Dementia in the Elderly

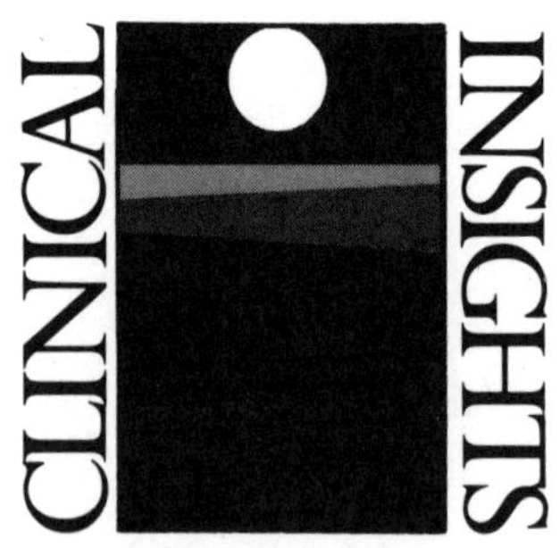

BIOLOGY AND TREATMENT OF

Dementia in the Elderly

Edited by
CHARLES A. SHAMOIAN, MD, PhD

*Associate Professor of Clinical Psychiatry and
Pharmacology, Cornell University Medical College; and
Director, Division of Geriatric Services, New York
Hospital–Cornell Medical Center*

AMERICAN PSYCHIATRIC PRESS, INC.
Washington, D.C.

Note: The authors have worked to ensure that all information in this book concerning drug dosages, schedules, and routes of administration is accurate at the time of publication and consistent with standards set by the U.S. Food and Drug Administration and the general medical community. As medical research and practice advance, however, therapeutic standards may change. For this reason and because human and mechanical errors sometimes occur, we recommend that readers follow the advice of a physician directly involved in their care or the care of a member of their family.

This monograph is based on material presented at the 136th Annual Meeting of the American Psychiatric Association. That meeting and this monograph are endeavors to share scientific findings and new ideas. The opinions expressed in this monograph are those of the individual authors and not necessarily those of the American Psychiatric Association.

Library of Congress Cataloging in Publication Data
Main entry under title:

Biology and treatment of dementia in the elderly.

(Clinical insights)
"Originally presented as part of a symposium . . . at the annual meeting of the American Psychiatric Association, held in New York City in May 1983"—P.
Includes bibliographies.
1. Alzheimer's disease—Congresses. I. Shamoian, Charles A. II. American Psychiatric Association. III. Series. [DNLM: 1. Dementia, Senile—Physiopathology—Congresses. 2. Dementia, Senile—Therapy—Congresses. WT 150 B615 1983]
RC523.B57 1984   618.97'68983   84-6226
ISBN 0-88048-051-3 (pbk.)

Printed in the U.S.A.

Contents

Contributors

George S. Alexopoulos, MD

Assistant Professor of Psychiatry, Cornell University Medical College; and Division of Geriatric Services, New York Hospital–Cornell Medical Center, Westchester Division

Ravi Anand, MD

Clinical Investigator, Geriatric Study and Treatment Program, New York University Medical Center

Jeffrey Borenstein, BA

Geriatric Study and Treatment Program, New York University Medical Center

John C. S. Breitner, MD

Assistant Professor of Psychiatry, The Johns Hopkins University School of Medicine; and Medical Director, Community Psychiatry Program, Baltimore City Hospital

Catharine Buttinger, MD

Clinical Investigator, Geriatric Study and Treatment Program, New York University Medical Center

Mony De Leon, EdD

Neuroscientist, Geriatric Study and Treatment Program, New York University Medical Center

Steven Ferris, MD

Executive Director, Geriatric Study and Treatment Program, New York University Medical Center

Marshall Folstein, MD

Associate Professor of Psychiatry and Medicine, The Johns Hopkins University School of Medicine; and Director, Division of General Hospital Psychiatry, The Johns Hopkins Hospital

TSU-KER FU, PHD

Psychogeriatric Unit, West Los Angeles VA Medical Center; and Department of Psychiatry and Biobehavioral Sciences, University of California, Los Angeles

JAMES A. HAYCOX, MD

Clinical Assistant Professor of Psychiatry, Cornell University Medical College; and Director, Psychiatric Services, Burke Rehabilitation Center

LISSY F. JARVIK, MD, PHD

Psychogeriatric Unit, West Los Angeles VA Medical Center; and Department of Psychiatry and Biobehavioral Sciences, University of California, Los Angeles

JOHN O. KESSLER, PHD

Physics Department, University of Arizona

KENNETH W. LIEBERMAN, PHD

Assistant Professor of Psychiatry and Biochemistry, Cornell University Medical College; and Payne Whitney Psychiatric Clinic

STEVEN S. MATSUYAMA, PHD

Psychogeriatric Unit, West Los Angeles VA Medical Center; and Department of Psychiatry and Biobehavioral Sciences, University of California, Los Angeles

DIANE POWELL, MD

Intern in Psychiatry and Medicine, Baltimore City Hospital

MURRAY RASKIND, MD

Associate Professor, Department of Psychiatry and Behavioral Sciences, University of Washington; and Director, Geriatric Research, Education, and Clinical Center, Seattle/American Lake VA Medical Centers

BARRY REISBERG, MD

Clinical Director, Geriatric Study and Treatment Program, New York University Medical Center

CHARLES A. SHAMOIAN, MD, PHD

Associate Professor of Clinical Psychiatry and Pharmacology, Cornell University Medical College; and Director, Division of Geriatric Services, New York Hospital–Cornell Medical Center

ELIA SINAIKO, PHD

Behavioral Biostatistician, Geriatric Study and Treatment Program, New York University Medical Center

Joe E. Thornton, MD

Laboratory of Clinical Psychopharmacology and Psychophysiology, VA Medical Center, Palo Alto; and Department of Psychiatry and Behavioral Sciences, Stanford University School of Medicine

Jared E. Tinklenberg, MD

Laboratory of Clinical Psychopharmacology and Psychophysiology, VA Medical Center, Palo Alto; and Department of Psychiatry and Behavioral Sciences, Stanford University School of Medicine

Jerome A. Yesavage, MD

Laboratory of Clinical Psychopharmacology and Psychophysiology, VA Medical Center, Palo Alto; and Department of Psychiatry and Behavioral Sciences, Stanford University School of Medicine

Robert C. Young, MD

Assistant Professor of Psychiatry, Cornell University Medical College; and Division of Geriatric Services, New York Hospital–Cornell Medical Center, Westchester Division

Introduction

The elderly now constitute approximately 12 percent of the general population in the United States. In another 50 years the aged will account for 18 to 20 percent of the population. This represents in absolute numbers an increase of elderly persons from approximately 24 million to almost 51 million (Plum 1979). The increase is projected to occur primarily in the old-old group, over the age of 75 years. By the year 2000 almost 50 percent of the elderly will be 75 years old or older (Kane et al. 1980).

Although dementia may occur during virtually any phase of the life cycle, it occurs primarily during old age (Tomlinson 1977). With the major shifts in the population described, the prevalence of dementia in our society can easily be predicted to be on the increase. In fact, our society has already begun to experience the emotional and financial ravages of this syndrome. Although many of the dementias are treatable and reversible, by far the most common type is that of senile dementia of the Alzheimer's type (SDAT), which is referred to as primary degenerative dementia in DSM-III (Tomlinson 1977). To date, SDAT is a disorder of unknown etiology with no known unequivocal specific treatment. However, with the marked interest recently manifested in this disorder, our knowledge and understanding of the biology of SDAT are rapidly advancing. Consequently, this should lead to earlier detection and diagnosis of the illness and should result in rational treatment approaches.

This monograph highlights some of the current approaches to the biology, diagnosis, and treatment of SDAT. These chapters were originally presented as part of a symposium on "The Biology and Treatment of Dementia in the Elderly" at the annual meeting of the American Psychiatric Association, held in New York City in May 1983.

The first two chapters, written by Dr. James A. Haycox and by Dr. Barry Reisberg and colleagues, provide the researcher and clinician with standardized scales to accurately assess the elderly SDAT patient's cognitive and behavioral functions. Haycox's Behavioral Scale for Dementia "documents the present behavioral status of a given demented patient, and its serial use charts the progress of a demented patient." Reisberg et al. describe in detail the Brief Cognitive Rating Scale and the Global Determination Scale for Alzheimer's disease. These studies have immediate relevance not only to assessment but also to management and counseling.

Dr. Marshall Folstein and colleagues, in the third chapter, review their studies and those in the literature which suggest that in a subgroup of patients, Alzheimer's disease may be genetically transmitted. In these patients the disease is familial and is thought to be transmitted as an age-dependent autosomal dominant trait. From a variety of different perspectives, these findings have immense implications.

The fourth chapter, by Dr. Steven S. Matsuyama et al., addresses the issue of possible biological markers for identifying patients with SDAT. Although still in the preliminary stages, the philothermal-response technique described in this study offers the hope that it may be a diagnostic test for SDAT. Clearly this paper is an example of the novel approaches needed if we are to solve the riddle of this mystifying disorder.

Recently, the reduction of brain acetylcholine in SDAT has been emphasized (Barcus et al. 1982). However, cholinomimetic agents have not augmented memory functions significantly in patients with SDAT. Dr. George S. Alexopoulos et al., in the fifth chapter, have investigated the possibility that other neurotransmitters such as the monoamines may be involved in this process. As determined by platelet monoamine oxidase activity, the investigators suggest the possibility of different subgroups of demented patients with different clinical profiles or biochemical abnormalities.

In the sixth chapter, Dr. Jared R. Tinklenberg et al. review the role of neuropeptides in improving cognitive functions. These authors, although critical about the currently available data, are of the belief that future studies will more clearly define the role of neuropeptides in geriatric psychopharmacology.

The final chapter by Dr. Murray Raskind reviews the current studies, which have used REM latency, the dexamethasone suppression test, and computed tomography (CT scan) to separate depression and dementia. These two disorders, which have an overlap of many significant symptoms, frequently present the clinician with a diagnostic challenge. It is hoped that future studies will provide biological markers to clearly differentiate these two ravaging illnesses that are so common to the elderly.

The intent of this monograph is to provide the reader with a general overview of some of the current approaches to the study, primarily, of senile dementia of the Alzheimer's type, which until a few years ago was perceived as a black box. Now at last we can look into this box that has been so often referred to as the "death of the mind."

Charles A. Shamoian, M.D., Ph. D.

(*NOTE:* George Alexopoulos, M.D. [Chapter 5] is supported by Faculty Development Award in Geriatric Mental Health no. 1–T01 MH 17508-01 AG-21 from the National Institute of Mental Health.)

References

Barcus, RD, Dean RL, Beer B, et al: The cholinergic hypothesis of geriatric memory dysfunction. Science 217:408–417, 1982

Kane R, Solomon D, Beck J, et al: The future need for geriatric manpower in the United States. N Engl J Med 302:1327–1332, 1980

Plum, F: Dementia: an approaching epidemic. Nature 279:372–373, 1979

Tomlinson, BE: The pathology of dementia, in Dementia, 2nd ed. Edited by Wells, CS. Philadelphia, FA Davis Co, 1977

1

A Behavioral Scale for Dementia

James A. Haycox, M.D.

1

A Behavioral Scale for Dementia

There are many tests and scales for rating cognitive function, but few of them can register the changes in a demented patient beyond the early stages (Reding et al. 1981). Behavioral assessment can document loss of capacities that do not necessarily rest directly on cognitive factors, and more readily illuminates a complete range of behavior from normal to terminal dementia.

Blessed et al. (1968) published perhaps the best known of behavioral scales, utilized in their studies on dementia. A more recent behavioral scale developed in Sweden was published by Gotfries et al. (1982). The scale presented here is better suited than either of the others for use with patients in the United States. Its clinical vocabulary tends to avoid ambiguity and is easily learned; it also documents the present behavioral status of a given demented patient, and its serial use charts the progress of a demented patient. Finally, it provides a tool for the comparison of clinical management methods including medication trials.

Preliminary exploration of serial scoring of patients with this scale suggests that appreciable failure in the social interplay and attention and awareness categories (described below) is a strong predictor of a declining course. Further analysis of more comprehensive data should clarify other features of dementia.

Use of this scale can call attention to the development of

symptoms that might otherwise remain unnoticed. The best care of dementia at present is maximizing the adaptation of patients to their disabilities. Fruitful management and treatment follow from good planning, which certainly rests on accurate clinical understanding of the individual patient.

DEVELOPMENT

Patients suffering from moderate-to-severe dementia of the Alzheimer's type (DAT) were observed in a day hospital. They were scored using the behavioral scale of Blessed et al. (1968) along with 11 cognitive tests. Each patient, usually accompanied by family, was examined by a psychiatrist, an internist, a neurologist, and a social worker. Past medical records were reviewed, and a comprehensive battery of laboratory tests was performed. At a clinical conference examiners made the diagnoses, and where disagreements were not easily settled, note was made of exceptions, which were studied later (M. Reding, personal communication).

The day-hospital group established a list of symptoms of dementia in progressive order. Each patient's status was documented with this list. Global ranking of patients according to increasing disability confirmed the correctness of the progression of the list. The ratings were performed by the participant–observer method to avoid intruding on patients.

Eight categories of symptoms developed as the list was clarified and refined:

- Language and conversation
- Social interaction
- Attention and awareness
- Spatial orientation
- Motor coordination
- Bowel and bladder habits
- Eating and nutrition
- Dressing and grooming

As indicated in Figure 1, each category was divided into seven steps (0 to 6; i.e., normal to most deranged), and by this system a

Figure 1 The Dementia Behavior Scale (Reproduced by permission from *The Journal of Clinical Psychiatry* 45:23–24, 1984).

NAME: ________________________________ DATE: ____________

TOTAL: ____________________ RATER'S INITIALS: ________________

LANGUAGE-CONVERSATION

0 Conversational
1 Repeats self, searches for synonyms, reticent conversation
2 Circumlocution, white lies, mild vocabulary limitation, easily led in conversation, automatisms
3 Loses thread of thought, noticeable vocabulary loss
4 Less aware of mistakes, poor syntax and sequence, perseveration, neologisms
5 Parrots words, incoherent, uncomprehending, severe vocabulary limitation
6 Mute, unresponsive

SOCIAL INTERACTION

0 Assists, takes initiative
1 Active participant, follower
2 Bland participant, no longer empathic, loss of tact, withdrawn, clinging
3 Observer only, misidentifies close relatives, at times belligerent-defensive-suspicious
4 Out of step, poor recognition of persons, mistakes own reflection, at times menacing
5 Wanders, frequent catastrophic reaction (defiant, suspicious, combative)
6 Blank

ATTENTION-AWARENESS

0 Bright, responsive
1 Requires guidance, can't recall date
2 Shortened attention, can't recall day, easily distracted
3 Wandering attention, easily tires, very few pleasures
4 Distracted by illusions, picks at imaginary lint, misidentifies objects
5 Can be engaged sporadically and briefly
6 Oblivious

SPATIAL ORIENTATION

0 Oriented
1 Oriented to immediate locus only (can't get home)
2 Hesitant, loses things
3 Disoriented to place, hides things, pack rat
4 Body disorientations, can't seat self on chair, bodily illusions, oblivious to posture
5 Hallucinating
6 Totally lost

MOTOR COORDINATION

0 Fully coordinated
1 Underactive, responsive to commands
2 Poorly coordinated, slowly moving, stumbling
3 Occasionally requires manipulation, occasionally requires assistance
4 Involuntary movements interfere, immobile, neglect of one side, requires manipulation and assistance
5 Spastic, chin on chest, wheelchair for safety, maximum physical assistance
6 Unable to ambulate, limbs contracted

BOWEL AND BLADDER

0 Self-care
1 Asks to go, needs cues to locate toilet
2 Remindable, poor hygiene occasionally, forgets to flush
3 Regular supervision, requires assistance, occasionally wet
4 Occasional fecal incontinence
5 Unpredictable, control by enema, occasional diapers
6 Fully incontinent, full-time diapers, full-time catheter

EATING AND NUTRITION

0 Self-care, weight steady, can cook
1 Needs prompting to eat, history of weight loss, burns pots
2 Needs food cut up, wanders from table, can't cook at all
3 Improper use of utensils, uses fingers, slight weight gain
4 Voraciously interested in sweets, steals food, marked weight gain, marked weight loss
5 Must be fed, eats nonfood
6 Tube fed, dysphagic

DRESS AND GROOMING

0 Appropriate self-care, well groomed
1 Won't change, poorly groomed
2 Dirty, ill-kempt, inappropriate dress, food on face
3 Misuse of clothing, misidentification of clothes, wears other's clothes, needs clothes set out
4 Dresses with instructions and help, oblivious to grooming
5 Requires full assistance
6 Must be dressed, hospital gown

completely nondemented person would score a total of 0 and a completely demented person would score 48.

THE SCALE

Language and Conversation

This category addresses verbal interplay between people. The term *speech* was not chosen because it is too specifically tied to the utterance of words.

Score 0: A normal person is responsive and conversational.

Score 1: Slight failure is characterized by reluctance in initiating conversation and a tendency toward use of synonyms because memory for common words is failing. There is repetition of statements or questions to an irritating degree (see the discussion of intrusion in Fuld 1983).

Score 2: The next step shows overuse of automatic, jargonistic phrases; there are confabulations, white lies, and circumlocution due to more memory failure.

Score 3: With moderate vocabulary loss a patient will lose the thread of a thought while speaking.

Score 4: An unawareness of language deficits leads to use of neologisms. Patient shows verbal perseveration of phrases, words, or syllables (intrusion).

Score 5: There is severe vocabulary limitation (a dozen or so words remain) with incoherence in speech and incomprehension in conversation.

Score 6: A mute and unresponsive person.

Social Interaction

The observations in this category are intended to gauge a patient's reaction to other human beings.

Score 0: A normal person assists in social interaction and takes initiative. Limited only by personality, he or she moves with the flow of social life.

Score 1: If a person is disabled to a slight degree, initiative is faulty even in the presence of receptive and considerate people. At times this person may show a pathetic eagerness to comply, trying to appear normal.

Score 2: Later the patient is a bland participant: withdrawn and showing uncharacteristic loss of tact.

Score 3: At this stage the patient is an observer only, misidentifying close relatives (before misidentifying other people). He or she is sometimes suspicious, defensive, and belligerent.

Score 4: The patient has become socially out of step and unable to discriminate among people. On occasion because of confusion he or she may be menacing. The patient may mistake his or her reflection in the mirror as another person.

Score 5: The patient goes to pieces under stress (also called **catastrophic reaction** and **agony**). At this time the patient is defiant and combative.

Score 6: The patient is socially blank.

Attention and Awareness

This category refers to the ability of a person to notice life and reality around him, to be captured by it, and to attend to it. The question is: Are there things that can hold the person's interest? Orientation to time is examined in this division (i.e., awareness of the passage of time).

Score 0: A normal person who is neither tired nor ill is alert, bright, and responsive unless attention is fixed on a task, in which case he or she is absorbed in it.

Score 1: Mild disability means that things must be pointed out or they remain unnoticed. The date is lost as a marking point.

Score 2: Attention span is shortened and the day of the week is lost. The person's zest for the present is diminished and he or she is easily distracted from the present activity.

Score 3: The person's attention wanders; he or she tires easily and is apathetic about the past and does not reminisce.

Score 4: In this stage the patient may mistake patterns in clothing for lint. In bed he or she may pluck at the counterpane or brush at imaginary dust.

Score 5: The patient's attention can't be engaged reliably and sometimes not at all.

Score 6: The patient is oblivious to everything except pain.

Spatial Orientation

Normally, spatial orientation is somewhat variable. One might awaken as a guest in an unfamiliar room and wonder where one is for a moment. In general, however, we know where we are or are able to deduce it. We can, for instance, use a map.

Score 0: Full orientation.

Score 1: A slight disability means that a person is oriented to the inside of the room that is occupied and perhaps is able to find the way a few rooms beyond, but not to get home from two blocks away.

Score 2: The person is hesitant about where he or she is and where things are and incessantly loses things.

Score 3: The patient is disoriented in all surroundings. The patient hides things and accumulates small things in his or her pockets (pack-rat phenomenon).

Score 4: The patient tends to place himself or herself inaccurately in a chair or may miss it altogether. The patient may remain in the inaccurate position, oblivious to having taken an odd posture. The patient may have the illusion that he or she is carrying something in an empty hand.

Score 5: Hallucinations occur late in the illness, indicating that the patient is oriented to his or her own thought and seems content to exclude reality.

Score 6: Spatial orientation is totally lost.

Motor Coordination

Older people do not necessarily lose their physical grace. Arthritis and physical disabilities certainly will shape the body and its movements, but motor coordination remains.

Score 0: Full coordination.

Score 1: The person is underactive but responsive to commands.

Score 2: The patient moves slowly, with occasional stumbling and poor coordination of fine movements. There is clumsiness in tying shoes, perhaps.

Score 3: Occasionally the patient requires assistance or outright manipulation.

Score 4: The patient shows a tendency to immobility, perhaps neglect of one side. There may be involuntary movements that interfere with his or her intentions.

Score 5: There is spasticity requiring physical assistance. The patient is transported by wheelchair for safety.

Score 6: The patient is unable to ambulate; limbs are contracted.

Bowel and Bladder Habits

Competence in managing bathroom functions well is socially crucial. Those who care for the demented may discover to their surprise that bowel and bladder retraining is often accomplished in patients who have lost the capacity. It is less a neurologic problem than a psychologic one. A patient must regain control or predictability if possible, since this one factor may determine whether or not he or she can remain at home.

Score 0: Self-care.

Score 1: The person asks to go to the toilet but may need cues to locate it.

Score 2: Reminders are necessary for toileting because the patient does not recognize his or her own need. Hygiene is poor and the person will forget to flush the toilet.

Score 3: The patient requires regular supervision and assistance and will occasionally wet himself or herself.

Score 4: Occasional fecal incontinence.

Score 5: The patient is unpredictable, controlled with enema, and occasionally wears diapers for safety.

Score 6: The patient is doubly incontinent, and full-time diapers and/or full-time catheter are necessary.

Eating and Nutrition

If accurate observations can be made, a score in this category is sensitive and reliable in assessing the stage of dementia. The spread of scores covers the wide range of burning a pot on the stove to being unable to swallow food safely (end stage).

Score 0: Self-care is possible; body weight holds steady; the ability to cook is retained if it was ever present.

Score 1: History of weight loss. Poorly tended pots burn on the stove. Nutrition may be poor and the patient may need urging and supervision to eat a sufficient diet despite an apparently normal appetite.

Score 2: The patient can't cook at all, wanders from the table, and may require food to be cut up for manageability.

Score 3: The patient may use fingers to eat because he or she can't use knife, fork, and spoon. There may be a slight weight gain at this time.

Score 4: The patient shows voracious interest in sweets and may filch food. He or she may show either marked weight gain or marked weight loss.

Score 5: The patient cannot manage alone and must be fed. The patient may eat things that are not food—napkins, plants, or dirt.

Score 6: Dysphagia is present, which is life threatening. The patient may require tube feeding or gastrostomy.

Dressing and Grooming

A patient's appearance will determine how people react and may dictate whether or not people can enjoy being with the patient. Social presentability helps a family to decide to keep a patient at home. Most patients lose interest and capacity for good grooming early.

Score 0: Good self-care. Good grooming.

Score 1: The person is slightly careless in appearance with reluctance to change clothes and to have them cleaned.

Score 2: There is food on the patient's face; he or she is ill-kempt (dirty clothes and body). Choice of clothing may be inappropriate.

Score 3: The patient misuses clothing and misidentifies garments, may wear the clothes of others, and needs clothing set out in order to dress.

Score 4: The patient dresses with instructions and some help and is oblivious to grooming.

Score 5: The patient requires full assistance. He or she can participate in dressing but cannot do it alone.

Score 6: Patient cannot dress alone at all. Often for convenience the patient is dressed in a hospital gown.

VALIDATION OF THE SCALE

Reliability Between Raters

The six observers in the validation studies may be arranged into 15 different pairs for comparison with each other. Each observer had scored the same 16 patients. Correlations between the scores for each of the 15 pairs were calculated by the Pearson method. The mean ($\pm$ SEM) of correlation coefficients was .93 $\pm$ .02. The ratings were repeated 10 days later, and the mean correlation for the second rating was .91 $\pm$ .05. Correlating each individual rater's first set of ratings with the second set showed a mean correlation of .97 $\pm$ .02, indicating high individual consistency as well as high reliability between raters.

Validity of Clinical Judgment

The same six observers were asked to rank patients from most ill to least ill. Their behavioral ratings, which were done at about the same time, were arranged in ranked series. Spearman rank correlations showed a mean ($\pm$ SEM) correlation between test ranking and clinical ranking of .66 $\pm$ .10. A second time, the correlation was .68 $\pm$ .43.

Behavioral Scoring by Telephone

Telephone scoring of behavior (indirect) was compared to the direct interview method. One rater scored 12 day-hospital patients as she saw them in the day hospital. At the same time another rater scored them by calling their relatives at home. Pearson correlation between the two methods is .89 $\pm$ .06. The implication is that telephone follow-up can be reliable and is useful in follow-up of patients at a distance from the center.

Comparisons with Other Tests

Correlation was shown between this behavioral scale and the Behavioral Rating Scale described by Blessed at al. (1968), done at the same time ($r = .61$, $p = .01$), which in turn had correlated well with the finding of Alzheimer's disease at autopsy ($r = .64$, $p = .001$). Correlation with the Kahn–Goldfarb Mental Status Quotient (Kahn et al. 1960) was $r = .55$ ($p = .01$).

Training Required

New users of the scale have been asked to read the description of the test and then to score those patients whom they know. Some items require the report of family members. Scoring is best done by underlining present symptoms and then circling the score number most fairly representing the patient's current status in a given category. If the trainer scores two or three patients at the same time, it will bring to light any questions. An hour should be sufficient to train a person.

SUMMARY

1. A scoring sheet for behavioral abnormalities in demented patients has been developed and has proven useful in clinical practice.
2. Interrater reliability is high. Average correlation on total score between pairs of raters was $.90 \pm .05$.
3. Each rater was self-consistent. Tests performed 10 days apart by the same rater correlated, on the average, $.97 \pm .02$.
4. Ratings correlated well with global clinical judgment of severity of impairment. Rank correlation average was $.66 \pm .10$.
5. Direct behavioral rating of patients was closely correlated to behavioral rating done by telephone to patients' families ($r = .89 \pm .06$).
6. This scale correlated well with the scale of Blessed et al. (1968) ($r = .61$, $p = .01$).

References

Blessed G, Tomlinson B, Roth M: The association between quantitative measures of dementia and senile changes in the cerebral grey matter of elderly subjects. Br J Psychiatry 114:797–811, 1968.

Fuld P: Word intrusion as a diagnostic sign in Alzheimer's disease. Geriatric Medicine Today. 2(4):33–41, 1983.

Gotfries C, Brane G, Gullberg B et al: A new rating scale for dementia syndromes. Archives of Gerontology and Geriatrics 11:311–330, 1982.

Kahn RL, Goldfarb AT, Pollack M et al: Brief objective measures for the determination of mental status in the aged. Am J Psychiatry 117:326–329, 1960.

Reding M, Haycox J, Tweedy J: Assessment of functional impairment in the dementias. Age 4(4):145, 1981.

2

Clinical Assessments of Cognition in the Aged

Barry Reisberg, M.D.
Steven Ferris, M.D.
Ravi Anand, M.D.
Catharine Buttinger, M.D.
Jeffrey Borenstein, B.A.
Elia Sinaiko, Ph.D.
Mony de Leon, Ed.D.

2

Clinical Assessments of Cognition in the Aged

The advent of geriatric psychiatry and psychopharmacology in recent years necessitated the development of clinical instruments with which to assess drug effects. Consequently clinical instruments were developed and came into wide usage. The best known of the initial instruments developed were the Sandoz Clinical Assessment Geriatric (SCAG) scale (Shader et al. 1974); the various mental status questionnaires (Kahn et al. 1960; Pfeiffer 1975; Folstein et al. 1975; Jacobs et al. 1977); functional assessment measures (Lawton 1971); and at least one scale that combined mental status and functional assessments (Blessed et al. 1968). Each of these instruments has certain advantages and certain disadvantages.

One major common disadvantage is that these measures were designed prior to our very recently developed understanding of the nature of geriatric mental illness. For example, the investigations that resulted in our current belief that dementia in the elderly is associated with Alzheimer's-type neuropathology and clinical symptomatology in the majority of instances, and multi-infarct-type neuropathology and clinical symptomatology in most remaining cases were first published between 1966 and 1970 (Roth et al. 1966; Blessed et al. 1968; Tomlinson et al. 1968, 1970). Nascent official recognition within the research community of the implications of these findings did not come until 1974 (Hachinski et al. 1974). The psychiatric nomenclature was modified in accordance with these findings in 1980 (American Psychiatric Association 1980). Finally, what are apparently the first detailed case histories describing the clinical course of Alzheimer's disease—or, in psychiatric terminology, primary degenerative dementia (PDD)—were not published until 1981 (Reisberg 1981). In contrast, the Mental Status Questionnaire (MSQ) scale was first published in 1960 and the SCAG was published in 1974 and was developed somewhat prior to that date.

Hence the measures described above either attempt to cover a very broad range of pathology, as in the case of the SCAG, or are entirely nonspecific and limited in range, as in the case of the MSQ. Until recently, no clinical scale existed that was specifically designed to assess cognitive functioning in a comprehensive and graded fashion. (Technically, the mental status questionnaires are psychometric rather than clinical scales since they require all-or-none responses which do not permit the clinician to take into account the patient's background and milieu. However, the mental status assessments are instruments that can easily be utilized by clinicians.) Also needed were scales that are specifically designed to assess pathology in the major mental disorders of the senium, notably Alzheimer's disease or senile dementia of the Alzheimer's type (SDAT), which afflicts literally millions of persons in the developed nations.

THE BRIEF COGNITIVE RATING SCALE

The major mental disorders of the senium are senescent forgetfulness; Alzheimer's disease; multi-infarct dementia; geriatric affective disorder, particularly geriatric depression; involutional psychoses; idiopathic Parkinson's disease; chronic schizophrenia; and chronic toxic brain disease, secondary to alcohol and other toxins. These illnesses are associated with a limited number of behavioral and neurologic syndromes. Notably, these syndromes are (a) cognitive impairment; (b) depression and anxiety; (c) psychosis; and (d) specific neurological syndromes such as the extra-

Table 1 Brief Cognitive Rating Scale (BCRS)

Axis	Rating (Circle Highest Score)	Item
Axis I: Concentration and Calculating Ability	1	No objective or subjective evidence of deficit in concentration.
	2	Subjective decrement in concentration ability.
	3	Minor objective signs of poor concentration (e.g., on subtraction of serial 7s from 100).
	4	Definite concentration deficit for persons of their background (e.g., marked deficit on serial 7s; frequent deficit in subtraction of serial 4s from 40).
	5	Marked concentration deficit (e.g., giving months backwards or serial 2s from 20).
	6	Forgets the concentration task. Frequently begins to count forward when asked to count backwards from 10 by 1s.
	7	Marked difficulty counting forward to 10 by 1s.
Axis II: Recent Memory	1	No objective or subjective evidence of deficit in recent memory.
	2	Subjective impairment only (e.g., forgetting names more than formerly).
	3	Deficit in recall of specific events evident upon detailed questioning. No deficit in the recall of major recent events.
	4	Cannot recall major events of previous weekend or week. Scanty knowledge (not detailed) of current events, favorite TV shows, etc.
	5	Unsure of weather; may not know current president or current address.
	6	Occasional knowledge of some recent events. Little or no idea of current address, weather, etc.
	7	No knowledge of any recent events.
Axis III: Remote Memory	1	No subjective or objective impairment in past memory.
	2	Subjective impairment only. Can recall two or more primary school teachers.
	3	Some gaps in past memory upon detailed questioning. Able to recall at least one childhood teacher and/or one childhood friend.

Table 1 Brief Cognitive Rating Scale (BCRS) *(cont.)*

Axis	Rating (Circle Highest Score)	Item
	4	Clear-cut deficit. The spouse recalls more of the patient's past then the patient. Cannot recall childhood friends and/or teachers but knows the names of most schools attended. Confuses chronology in reciting personal history.
	5	Major past events sometimes not recalled (e.g., names of schools attended).
	6	Some residual memory of past (e.g., may recall country of birth or former occupation).
	7	No memory of past.
Axis IV: Orientation	1	No deficit in memory for time, place, identity of self or others.
	2	Subjective impairment only. Knows time to nearest hour, location.
	3	Any mistake in time - 2 hrs; day of week - 1 day; date - 3 days.
	4	Mistakes in month - 10 days or year - one month.
	5	Unsure of month and/or year and/or season; unsure of locale.
	6	No idea of date. Identifies spouse but may not recall name. Knows own name.
	7	Cannot identify spouse. May be unsure of personal identity.
Axis V: Functioning and Self-Care	1	No difficulty, either subjectively or objectively.
	2	Complains of forgetting location of objects. Subjective work difficulties
	3	Decreased job functioning evident to co-workers. Difficulty in traveling to new locations.
	4	Decreased ability to perform complex tasks (e.g., planning dinner for guests, handling finances, marketing, etc.).
	5	Requires assistance in choosing proper clothing.
	6	Requires assistance in feeding, and/or toileting, and/or bathing, and/or dressing.
	7	Requires constant assistance in all activities of daily life.

Note. Adapted from Reisberg et al. 1983a.

pyramidal syndrome (EPS). Excellent, brief, standardized clinical rating instruments exist which are specifically designed to assess three of these four syndromes. Specifically, these include the Hamilton scale for depression and anxiety (Hamilton 1960); the Brief Psychiatric Rating scale (BPRS) (Overall and Gorham 1962) for psychosis; and the Simpson-Angus scale for EPS (Simpson and Angus 1970), among others. No brief clinical rating scale existed that was specifically designed to assess the syndrome of cognitive decline. Since cognitive decline is either a notable (or *the* notable) feature of many of the geriatric mental illnesses enumerated above, it behooved clinicians and investigators to have an instrument specifically designed to assess this syndrome rapidly and comprehensively.

Accordingly, we have developed an instrument for the rapid and structured assessment of the clinical aspects of cognitive decline, regardless of etiology. This instrument is analogous to the Hamilton scale for the depressive syndrome and the BPRS for the syndrome of psychosis (i.e., it assesses the severity of a clinical syndrome and not any particular diagnostic entity). The instrument is known as the Brief Cognitive Rating Scale (BCRS) (Table 1). The BCRS assesses the magnitude of cognitive impairment on five clinical axes using specified criteria. The axes represented are (I) concentration and calculating ability, (II) recent memory, (III) remote memory, (IV) orientation, and (V) functioning and self-care. Items are scored from information obtained during a structured clinical interview conducted in the presence of a spouse or caregiver where possible. This interview procedure is particularly important in light of the denial that frequently accompanies moderate-to-severe memory loss (Reisberg et al., in press).

Each axis utilizes seven rating points that correspond to seven definable and distinguishable stages of cognitive functioning within each axis. The axes were designed so that patients with normal aging or SDAT show a fairly uniform magnitude of cognitive and functional ability on each of the concordant axes. The clinical characteristics of the ratings on each axis are also designed to coincide with each corresponding Global Deterioration

Scale (GDS) stage (Reisberg et al. 1982) in patients with normal aging and PDD (Reisberg and Ferris 1982).

We have attempted to assess the validity of these assumptions with respect to the design of the clinical axes, and also to obtain information on the validity of the axes, in initial investigations with 18 subjects (Reisberg et al. 1983a) and in further investigations utilizing the procedures described below.

Method

Fifty consecutive outpatients were studied: 25 men and 25 women. The mean ($\pm$ SD) age was 71.2 $\pm$ 7.01 years. These subjects consisted of controls (GDS stage 1) with average or superior cognitive function for their ages who demonstrated neither subjective nor objective evidence of cognitive deterioration ($n = 9$), subjects with very mild impairment (GDS stage 2) consistent with the generally benign symptomatology of normal aging ($n = 21$), subjects with mild cognitive deterioration (GDS stage 3) consistent with either age-associated decline or very early stage PDD ($n = 4$), and subjects with moderate-to-severe cognitive deterioration (GDS stage 4–6) consistent with PDD ($n = 16$). Patient evaluations were conducted by experienced geriatric clinicians who were not involved in the development of the clinical rating instruments. All subjects received extensive medical, psychiatric, neurologic, and neuroradiologic examinations prior to entry into the study. Subjects with factors that might contribute to cognitive impairment other than normal aging or PDD were excluded from participation.

All study subjects received psychometric and mental status evaluations as well as clinical assessments. The psychometric evaluations were conducted by psychologists independently of the clinical assessments. The specific evaluations utilized consisted of the five subtests of the Guild Memory Test (Gilbert et al. 1968; Gilbert and Levee 1971) and the WAIS vocabulary subtest, digit symbol substitution task, and forward and backward digit span (Wechsler 1945). The subjects also received a brief Mental Status Questionnaire as described by Kahn et al. (1960).

Table 2   BCRS: Pearson Correlations ($p < .001$) with Independent Psychometric and Mental Status Questionnaire Assessments ($N = 50$)

Assessment Method	Axis I	Axis II	Axis III	Axis IV	Axis V	BCRS Total Score
Guild Test Battery						
(a) Paragraph, initial recall	.69	.74	.64	.69	.67	.72
(b) Paragraph, delayed recall	.68	.70	.61	.69	.68	.71
(c) Paired associate recall, initial	.60	.63	.51	.62	.62	.63
(d) Paired associate recall, delayed	.57	.60	.48	.56	.59	.59
(e) Designs	.65	.71	.59	.66	.69	.70
Combined Guild score	.72	.76	.64	.72	.72	.75
WAIS Vocabulary (raw scores)	.72	.78	.74	.68	.69	.76
Digit Symbol Substitution Test	.76	.78	.71	.71	.73	.78
Digit Span						
Forward	.64	.71	.71	.68	.66	.72
Backward	.69	.77	.71	.71	.65	.74
Total	.73	.84	.78	.77	.68	.79
Mental Status Questionnaire scores	.72	.75	.68	.78	.72	.77

To evaluate the validity of the clinical axes, Pearson correlation coefficients were computed between scores on each of the clinical axes and performance on the psychometric tests and Mental Status Questionnaire. In order to evaluate the concordance of deficit across the five clinical axes, the intercorrelations among the axis scores were examined.

Results

The relationships obtained between clinical assessments and the independently obtained psychometric and mental status evaluations can be seen in Table 2. All correlations were statistically significant ($p < .001$) and ranged from .51 to .84. The correlations with combined psychometric assessments (total Guild scores and digit span total scores) tended to be higher than the correlations with any individual psychometric assessment measures. Similarly, the correlations obtained for the WAIS vocabulary scores, the digit symbol substitution test scores, and Mental Status Ques-

Table 3 Pearson Intercorrelations ($p < .001$) of BCRS Axes ($N = 50$)

	Axis I	Axis II	Axis III	Axis IV	Axis V
Axis I	. . .	.91	.89	.91	.88
Axis II	. . .	. . .	.88	.94	.90
Axis III	. . .	. . .	. . .	.88	.83
Axis IV	. . .	. . .	. . .	. . .	.94
BCRS Total Scores	.96	.97	.94	.97	.95
GDS Scores	.90	.94	.87	.94	.91

tionnaire scores were of comparable magnitude to the combined psychometric assessments. Hence, the clinical axes correlated most strongly with combined memory test scores, general assessment of language ability, coupled psychomotor interaction, and global mental status.

Interrelationships among the five clinical axes ranged between .83 and .94 (see Table 3). All individual axis correlations with total scores for the five axes combined and with GDS scores were .90 or greater.

Discussion

These findings indicate that each of the clinical axes is consistently and significantly correlated with the magnitude of psychometrically determined cognitive impairment in subjects with age-associated cognitive decline and PDD. These correlations appear to be particularly strong for combined and relatively "global" psychometric assessments. Furthermore, as intended in the design of the clinical assessments, the clinical axes do indeed show strong concordance over the range of normal aging and PDD. The magnitude of these interrelationships is sufficiently great as to raise the question of redundancy and whether multiple clinical modalities (or axes) are needed.

There are several reasons why multiple clinical assessments are desirable. These include (a) the utility of such measures in confirming the diagnosis and in differential diagnosis of normal age-associated cognitive changes and primary degenerative dementia; (b) the utility of detailed assessments in sensitively and accurately gauging the value of putative treatment interventions;

and (c) the utility of detailed assessments as research tools in increasing our understanding of the clinical characteristics and evolution of the disorder.

The clinical axes are specifically designed to parallel and to be concordant with the unique and characteristic clinical syndrome of age-associated cognitive decline and PDD. Cognitive impairment associated with other etiologies such as geriatric depression, multi-infarct dementia, or alcoholism would be expected to show different or less concordant patterns on the clinical axes. For example, patients with geriatric depression may show relatively greater impairment on the concentration assessments (Axis I), in comparison with recent memory (Axis II). If this hypothesis is confirmed, then increased scores on the concentration axis in comparison to the recent-memory axis, for example, might alert clinicians to the possible presence of depression. Conversely, uniform scores on the various clinical axes can serve to help confirm a clinician's diagnosis of PDD. These brief procedures can be readily performed in an office setting and provide objective criteria which can be of value in the interchange of clinical information (Reisberg 1982).

The ordinal clinical assessments may also be useful in the succinct staging of age-associated cognitive decline and PDD. With respect to succinct staging, Axis V, reflecting functioning and self-care, may be particularly useful; this aspect of Axis V will be discussed in greater detail in a subsequent section of this chapter.

THE GLOBAL DETERIORATION SCALE (GDS) FOR ALZHEIMER'S DISEASE

The clinical symptomatology of persons with cognitive decline consistent with normal aging or SDAT varies depending upon the magnitude or *stage* of cognitive impairment. Within each stage, symptomatology is fairly consistent. The global clinical characteristics of each stage of cognition in normal aged persons and in those with mild-to-severe Alzheimer's disease can be seen in the Global Deterioration Scale for Age-Associated Cognitive Decline and Alzheimer's Disease, which is described in Table 4.

Previous investigations have revealed strong, significant relationships between progressive decline on these global clinical parameters and independent behavioral (Reisberg et al. 1982a, Reisbergt et al. 1982b), neuroradiologic (de Leon et al. 1979, 1980, 1983a, 1983b), neurometabolic (Ferris et al. 1980; de Leon et al. 1983a, 1983b, 1983c), and neuroimmunologic (Nandy et al. 1981) assessments in subjects with normal aging and progressive PDD.

Initial prognostic concomitants of these global clinical stages of normal aging and SDAT in community-residing outpatients have also recently been published (Reisberg et al. 1983b). These initial prospective longitudinal investigations revealed that after a mean follow-up interval of approximately 27 months, all 16 forgetfulness-phase patients (GDS stage 2) who were followed remained alive, healthy, and community residing and were essentially no worse on clinical cognitive or functional assessments. Hence this stage appeared to truly represent that of benign senescent forgetfulness.

Fourteen early-confusional-phase outpatients (GDS stage 3) followed over this interval also all remained alive, healthy, and in the community at follow-up. However, as a group these subjects declined at a significantly faster rate on clinical cognizance parameters than the forgetfulness-phase subjects. Hence, this early confusional phase may represent a "borderline" stage between the truly benign symptoms of normal aging and the more malignant symptomatology of PDD. However, it should be noted that although these early-confusional-phase subjects declined at a significantly greater rate than the forgetfulness-phase subjects as a group, at least half of the 14 subjects who were followed individually showed no decline over the interval.

In the initial longitudinal investigation, the late confusional phase (GDS stage 4) appeared to herald a much more malignant prognosis for most subjects. Of 11 individuals followed two were deceased, one was in a nursing home, and eight remained in the community. Of this latter group, half were worse clinically, and half appeared not to have declined. Clearly, none of these subjects improved. Hence, this late confusional phase can probably be said

Table 4 Global Deterioration Scale (GDS) for Age-Associated Cognitive Decline and Alzheimer's Disease (Reisberg et al. 1982b)

GDS Stage	Clinical Phase	Clincal Characteristics
1 No cognitive decline	Normal	No subjective complaints of memory deficit. No memory deficit evident on clinical interview.
2 Very mild cognitive decline	Forgetfulness	Subjective complaints of memory deficit, most frequently in following areas: (a) forgetting where one has placed familiar objects; (b) forgetting names one formerly knew well. No objective evidence of memory deficit on clinical interview. No objective deficits in employment or social situations. Appropriate concern with respect to symptomatology.
3 Mild cognitive decline	Early confusional	Earliest clear-cut deficits. Manifestations in more than one of the following areas: (a) patient may have gotten lost when traveling to an unfamiliar location; (b) co-workers become aware of patient's relatively poor performance; (c) word and name finding deficits become evident to intimates; (d) patient may read a passage or a book and retain relatively little material; (e) patient may demonstrate decreased facility in remembering names upon introduction to new people; (f) patient may have lost or misplaced an object of value; (g) concentration deficit may be evident on clinical testing. Objective evidence of memory deficit obtained only with an intensive interview conducted by a trained geriatric psychiatrist. Decreased performance in demanding employment and social settings. Denial begins to become manifest in patient. Mild to moderate anxiety accompanies symptoms.
4 Moderate cognitive decline	Late confusional	Clear-cut deficit on careful clinical interview. Deficit manifest in following areas: (a) decreased knowledge of current and recent events; (b) may exhibit some deficit in memory of one's personal history; (c) concentration deficit elicited on serial subtractions; (d) decreased ability to travel, handle finances, etc. Frequently no deficit in following areas: (a) orientation to time and person; (b) recognition of familiar persons and faces; (c) ability to travel to familiar locations. Inability to perform complex tasks. Denial is dominant defense mechanism. Flattening of affect and withdrawal from challenging situations occur.

5 Moderately severe decline	Early dementia	Patient can no longer survive without some assistance. Patient is unable during interview to recall a major relevant aspect of their current lives: e.g., their address or telephone number of many years, the names of close members of their family (such as grandchildren), the name of the high school or college from which they graduated. Frequently some disorientation to time (date, day of week, season, etc.) or to place. An educated person may have difficulty counting back from 40 by 4s or from 20 by 2s. Persons at this stage retain knowledge of many major facts regarding themselves and others. They invariably know their own names and generally know their spouses and children's names. They require no assistance with toileting or eating, but may have some difficulty choosing the proper clothing to wear.
6 Severe cognitive decline	Middle dementia	May occasionally forget the name of the spouse upon whom they are entirely dependent for survival. Will be largely unaware of all recent events and experiences in their lives. Retain some knowledge of their past lives but this is very sketchy. Generally unaware of their surroundings, the year, the season, etc. May have difficulty counting from 10, both backward and sometimes forward. Will require some assistance with activities of daily living, e.g., may become incontinent, will require travel assistance but occasionally will display ability to travel to familiar locations. Diurnal rhythm frequently disturbed. Almost always recall their own name. Frequently continue to be able to distinguish familiar from unfamiliar persons in their environment. Personality and emotional changes occur. These are quite variable and include: (a) delusional behavior, e.g., patients may accuse their spouse of being an impostor; may talk to imaginary figures in the environment, or to their own reflection in the mirror; (b) obsessive symptoms, e.g., person may continually repeat simple cleaning activities; (c) anxiety symptoms, agitation, and even previously nonexistent violent behavior may occur; (d) cognitive abulia, i.e., loss of willpower because an individual cannot carry a thought long enough to determine a purposeful course of action.
7 Very severe cognitive decline	Late dementia	All verbal abilities are lost. Frequently there is no speech at all—only grunting. Incontinent of urine; requires assistance toileting and feeding. Lose basic psychomotor skills, e.g., ability to walk. The brain appears to no longer be able to tell the body what to do. Generalized and cortical neurologic signs and symptoms.

to represent early SDAT, defined in terms of continued and gradual decline, for the majority of patients with this symptomatology.

In the initial prognostic studies described above, six individuals with early-dementia-phase symptoms (GDS stage 5) were followed. One of these was deceased, two were in nursing homes, and three were in the community, albeit clinically deteriorated at the time of follow-up. Hence, all of the early-dementia-phase subjects who were followed appeared to have symptomatology consistent with SDAT.

Longitudinal investigations of aging and dementia subgroups have continued in our laboratory, and more extensive prognostic data is presently available and can be seen in Table 5. Summarized, these investigations lead to the following conclusions:

(1) Forgetfulness-phase (GDS stage 2) symptomatology is indeed benign.

(2) The early confusional phase (GDS stage 3) represents a borderline condition between normal aging and Alzheimer's disease. Although the great majority of persons with these symptoms do not demonstrate further decline over an interval of approximately four years, somewhat less than 10 percent of these individuals do worsen sufficiently as to result in institutionalization or even death.

(3) The late confusional phase (GDS stage 4) represents the earliest stage of Alzheimer's disease. All of these subjects have declined notably from their premorbid level of functioning. None of these patients regain their former cognitive abilities. However, after an interval of approximately four years, roughly a quarter of these patients are not notably worsened clinically, while another quarter are notably worse, but still reside in the community. Our results indicate that a quarter of late-confusional-phase subjects require institutionalization over the subsequent four-year interval and the final quartile are deceased.

(4) The early dementia phase (GDS stage 5) is the second stage of Alzheimer's disease. Although, in accordance with our conceptualizations with respect to decline in so-called degenerative

Table 5 Aging and Dementia: Longitudinal Course of Community-Residing Subgroups

Clinical Status at Baseline	N	Age (mean ± SD years)	Sex	Follow-up Interval (mean ± SD days)	Follow-up Status
Forgetfulness Phase (GDS 2)	40	68.80 ± 5.29	21 M 19 F	1252 ± 151	40 Community Residing 2 Clinically Worsened* 38 Clinically Unchanged
Early Confusional Phase (GDS 3)	32	71.09 ± 6.79	16 M 16 F	1310 ± 181	30 Community Residing 3 Clinically Improved 3 Clinically Worsened 24 Clinically Unchanged 1 Institutionalized† 1 Deceased
Late Confusional Phase (GDS 4)	22	72.32 ± 5.75	4 M 18 F	1342 ± 212	10 Community Residing 4 Clinically Worsened 6 Clinically Unchanged 6 Institutionalized 6 Deceased
Early Dementia Phase (GDS 5)	6	72.33 ± 7.37	3 M 3 F	1505 ± 242	3 Community Residing 1 Clinically Worsened 2 Clinically Unchanged 2 Institutionalized 1 Deceased
Middle Dementia Phase (GDS 6)	6	72.50 ± 3.83	5 M 1 F	1523 ± 201	0 Community Residing 4 Institutionalized 2 Deceased

*Clinical change is defined as a change of 2 or greater in GDS scores from baseline.
†In nursing homes.

dementia, the majority of these patients do show further decline, it is worthy of note that some of these early-dementia-phase patients are not notably worsened after an interval of approximately four years.

(5) The middle dementia phase (GDS stage 6) is the third stage of Alzheimer's disease. Approximately a third of these patients are deceased after a four-year interval. The remaining two-thirds of these patients were in nursing homes when followed-up after a four-year interval. None of these patients whom we followed survived in a community setting over the four-year interval.

FUNCTIONAL ASSESSMENT STAGING OF ALZHEIMER'S DISEASE

Recent work has indicated that functionally one can distinguish at least 15 distinct progressive stages in the continuum from normal aging to the end stages of Alzheimer's disease. These functional assessment stages (FAST) represent an expansion of Axis V of the BCRS and hence can be divided into seven major concordant stages with the GDS, as well as into further subdivisions, as seen in Table 6.

Observations reveal that in uncomplicated SDAT these FAST stages proceed in an ordinal fashion (Reisberg et al., in press). Hence, SDAT patients who have difficulty marketing and handling their finances (FAST stage 4) are always beyond the point at which they would demonstrate evident deficit in demanding employment settings (FAST stage 3). Similarly, patients with uncomplicated SDAT always lose the ability to select their clothing properly (FAST stage 5) after they have lost the ability to market and handle their finances (FAST stage 4). Furthermore, SDAT patients always lose the ability to dress themselves properly (FAST stage 6a) after they are no longer capable of choosing their clothing properly (FAST stage 5).

In the sixth and seventh global stages, corresponding to the middle and late dementia phases, five distinct, functional sub-stages are identifiable. Distinctions between these substages are

Table 6 Functional Assessment Stages (FAST) in Normal Aging and Alzheimer's Disease

Global Deterioration Scale	Clinical Phase	FAST Characteristics
1, No cognitive decline	Normal	No functional decrement—either subjectively or objectively—manifest.
2, Very mild cognitive decline	Forgetfulness	Complains of forgetting location of objects; subjective work difficulties.
3, Mild cognitive decline	Early Confusional	Decreased functioning in demanding employment settings evident to co-workers; difficulty in traveling to new locations.
4, Moderate cognitive decline	Late Confusional	Decreased ability to perform complex tasks such as planning dinner for guests, handling finances, and marketing.
5, Moderately severe cognitive decline	Early Dementia	Requires assistance in choosing proper clothing; may require coaxing to bathe properly.
6, Severe cognitive decline	Middle Dementia	(a) Difficulty putting on clothing properly (b) Requires assistance bathing; may develop fear of bathing (c) Inability to handle mechanics of toileting (d) Urinary incontinence (e) Fecal incontinence
7, Very severe cognitive decline	Late Dementia	(a) Ability to speak limited to one to five words (b) All intelligible vocabulary lost (c) All motoric abilities lost (d) Stupor (e) Comatose

relatively subtle. Nevertheless, in the majority of Alzheimer's patients, functional progression appears to be ordinal for the substages as well as for the more distinct integer stages.

The recognition of these stages represents a considerable advance in our understanding of Alzheimer's disease since they enable clinicians and scientists to accurately quantify, in a readily comprehensible manner, the precise magnitude of impairment in Alzheimer's disease much more readily and accurately than previously. They also represent an advance in enabling clinicians to accurately and differentially diagnose Alzheimer's disease.

For example, if a patient with cognitive impairment of gradual onset loses the ability to walk (functional stage 7c) but the patient is still capable of articulating words, then an etiologic or confounding illness such as central nervous system neoplastic disease or stroke becomes much more likely to be the origin of the patient's impairment than Alzheimer's disease. Similarly, patients with so-called depressive pseudodementia may lose the ability to dress themselves but still be capable of choosing the proper clothing to wear. An Alzheimer's patient always loses the ability to choose clothing properly (functional stage 5) before losing the ability to put on clothing properly (functional stage 6a). Hence, the ordinal progression of functional loss in normal aging and SDAT provides a particularly useful tool for both the diagnosis and differential diagnosis of the age-associated cognitive disorders.

THE MINI-MENTAL STATE SCALE: UTILITY IN ALZHEIMER'S DISEASE

As discussed in the introduction to this chapter, a variety of instruments that are capable of assessing the magnitude of dementia symptomatology, irrespective of the etiology of the dementia, have been available for several years. One of the most useful and widely utilized of these instruments is the Mini-Mental State (MMS) scale. The advent of specific assessment instruments for grading the severity of symptomatology in normal aging and SDAT enables us to define the following MMS concomitants of normal aging and SDAT: (a) the MMS range at which true SDAT begins; (b) the MMS range of the borderline stage between that of normal aging and true SDAT; (c) the MMS range corresponding to the benign symptomatology of senescent forgetfulness; and (d) the stage in the progression of SDAT in which patients begin to score 0 on the MMS scales, and hence the stage at which this parameter is no longer of real utility in the assessment of Alzheimer's patients.

Preliminary answers to each of the above questions can be seen in Table 7. Table 7 demonstrates that the relationship between MMS scores and GDS scores in subjects with normal aging and

Table 7 Relationships Between Global Deterioration Score (GDS) Assignments and Mini-Mental Status (MMS) Scores in 40 Consecutive Subjects with Cognitive Function Consistent with Normal Aging or PDD (Dementia of the Alzheimer's Type)

GDS	Subjects (n)*	MMS (range)
2	4	25–30
3	7	20–27
4	8	16–23
5	11	10–19
6	10	0–12
Total	40	0–30

Note. Pearson correlation between GDS scores and MMS scores, −.924. GDS is described in Reisberg et al. 1982b; MMS is described in Folstein et al. 1975.
*10 male and 30 female; mean ± SD age, 70.73 ± 8.0 years (range, 51–83 years).

SDAT is quite strong ($r = -0.92$, *p.* $< .0001$). In subjects with uncomplicated SDAT, for whom other possible etiologic factors that are capable of producing dementia have been eliminated, the range of MMS scores corresponding to the late confusional phase (GDS stage 4), and hence early SDAT, is 16–23. Consequently, subjects with MMS scores greater than 23 cannot be said to have true Alzheimer's disease. Subjects with MMS scores from 25–30 may have symptomatology consistent with the benign prognosis of the forgetfulness phase (GDS stage 2). The borderline between early SDAT and benign senescent forgetfulness occurs in the MMS range of 20–27, corresponding to the early confusional phase (GDS stage 3). It may be possible for clinicians to further differentiate these patients with respect to prognostic classification using the clinical criteria described in Table 4.

Subjects with middle-dementia-phase symptomatology corresponding to GDS scores of 6 may score 0 on MMS assessments. Independent studies indicate that even SDAT patients at FAST stage 6a may score 0 on the MMS. Hence, clinically one can distinguish 10 functional stages of SDAT (6a–6e and 7a–7e) in which the MMS has little or no utility in assessing the magnitude of SDAT symptomatology. For these reasons the MMS is not very useful as a sole criterion in the study of patients with severe SDAT or in longitudinal studies of SDAT.

CONCLUSION

In the past few years considerable advances have been made in the field of clinical assessment of cognition in the aged. Clinical instruments, such as the Brief Cognitive Rating Scale, that are capable of sensitively assessing cognitive functioning regardless of etiology have been developed. A specific instrument for assessing the magnitude of deterioration in normal aging and SDAT, the Global Deterioration scale for Alzheimer's disease, has also been developed and validated. Prognostic concomitants of the GDS stages have been studied, which enable us to accurately describe the stages compatible with normal aging, early SDAT, and even a generally benign borderline stage. Functional criteria have been exploited in order to better define the later stages of SDAT, in which psychometric test measures and mental status assessment measures are no longer of utility. Finally, the relationship between recently developed assessments specific to SDAT symptomatology (such as the GDS and the FAST) and more general clinical assessments of dementia of diverse etiology are being defined.

Collectively, these advances have immediate relevance with respect to office management counseling and assessment, as well as with respect to the choice of measures and of patient populations for pharmacologic treatment trials.

References

American Psychiatric Association: Diagnostic and Statistical Manual of Mental Disorders, 3rd ed. Washington DC, American Psychiatric Association, 1980, p. 126

Blessed G, Tomlinson BE, Roth M: The association between quantitative measures of dementia and senile changes in the cerebral grey matter of elderly subjects. Br J Psychiatry 114:797–811, 1968

de Leon MJ, Ferris SH, Blau I, et al: Correlations between CT changes and behavioral deficits in senile dementia. Lancet 2:859, 1979 de Leon MJ, Ferris SH, George AE, et al: Computed tomography evaluations of brain–behavior relationships in senile dementia of the Alzheimer's type. Neurobiol Aging 1:69–79, 1980

de Leon MJ, George AE, Ferris SH, et al: Regional correlation of PET and CT in senile dementia of the Alzheimer's type. AJNR 4:553–556, 1983a

de Leon MJ, Ferris SH, George AE, et al: Computed tomography and positron emission transaxial tomography evaluations of normal aging and Alzheimer's disease. Journal of Cerebral Blood Flow and Metabolism 3:391–394, 1983b

de Leon MJ, Ferris SH, George AE, et al: Positron emission tomography studies of aging and Alzheimer's disease. AJNR 4:568–571, 1983c

Ferris SH, de Leon MH, Wolf AP, et al: Positron emission tomography in the study of aging and senile dementia. Neurobiol Aging 1:127–131, 1980

Folstein MF, Folstein SE, McHugh PR: "Mini-Mental state": a practical method for grading the cognitive state of patients for the clinician. J Psychiatr Res 12:189–198, 1975

Gilbert JG, Levee RF: Patterns of declining memory. J Gerontol 26:70, 1971

Gilbert JG, Levee RF, Catalano FL: A preliminary report on a new memory scale. Percept Mot Skills 27:277, 1968

Hachinski VC, Lassen NA, Marshall J: Multi-infarct dementia: a cause of mental deterioration in the elderly. Lancet 2:207–209, 1974

Hamilton M: A rating scale for depression. J Neurol Neurosurg Psychiatry 23:56–62, 1960

Jacobs JW, Bernhard MR, Delgado A, Strain JF: Screening for organic mental syndromes in the mentally ill. Ann Intern Med 80:40–46, 1977

Kahn RL, Goldfarb AI, Pollack M, et al: Brief objective measures for the determination of mental status in the aged. Am J Psychiatry 117:326–328, 1960

Lawton MP: The functional assessment of elderly people. J Am Geriatr Soc 19:465–481, 1971

Nandy K, Reisberg B, Ferris SH, et al: Brain reactive antibodies and progressive cognitive decline in the aged (abstr). Journal of the American Aging Association 4:145, 1981

Overall JE, Gorham DR: The brief psychiatric rating scale. Psychol Rep 10:799–812, 1962

Pfeiffer EA: Short portable mental status questionnaire for the assessment of organic brain deficit in the elderly. J Am Geriatr Soc 23:433–441, 1975

Reisberg B: Brain Failure: An Introduction to Current Concepts of Senility. New York, The Free Press/Macmillan, 1981, pp 81–122

Reisberg B: The office management of primary degenerative dementia. Psychiatric Annals 12:631, 1982

Reisberg B, Ferris SH: Diagnosis and assessment of the older patient. Hosp Community Psychiatry 33:104, 1982

Reisberg B, Ferris SH, Crook T: Signs, symptoms, and course of age-associated cognitive decline, in Alzheimer's Disease: A Report of Progress in Research. Edited by Corkin S, Davis KL, Growdon JH, et al. New York, Raven Press, 1982a, pp 177–181

Reisberg B, Ferris SH, de Leon MJ, et al: The global deterioration scale (GDS): an instrument for the assessment of primary degenerative dementia (PDD). Am J Psychiatry 139:1136–1139, 1982b

Reisberg B, Schneck MK, Ferris SH, et al: The brief cognitive rating scale (BCRS): findings in primary degenerative dementia (PDD). Psychopharmacol Bull 19:47–50, 1983a

Reisberg B, Shulman E, Ferris SH, et al: Clinical assessments of age-associated cognitive decline and primary degenerative dementia: prognostic concomitants. Psychopharmacol Bull 19:734–739, 1983b

Reisberg B, Gordon B, McCarthy M, et al: Clinical symptoms accompanying progressive cognitive decline and Alzheimer's disease: relationship to denial and ability to give informed consent. In Senile Dementia of the Alzheimer's Type and Related Disorders: Ethical and Legal Issues Related to Informed Consent. Edited by Melnick VL, Dubler N. Clifton, NJ, Humana Press (in press)

Reisberg G, Ferris SH, Anad R, et al: Fuctional staging of dementia of the Alzheimer's type. Ann NY Acad Sci. (in press)

Roth M, Tomlinson BE, Blessed G: Correlation between scores for dementia and counts of "senile plaques" in cerebral grey matter of elderly subjects. Nature 209:109, 1966

Shader RI, Harmatz AB, Salzman CA: A new scale for clinical assessment in geriatric populations: Sandoz-Clinical Assessment Geriatric (SCAG). J Am Geriatr Soc 22:107–113, 1974

Simpson GM, Angus JWS: A rating scale for extrapyramidal side effects. Acta Psychiatr Scand [Suppl] 212:11–19, 1970

Tomlinson BE, Blessed G, Roth M: Observations on the brains of non-demented old people. J Neurol Sci 7:331–356, 1968

Tomlinson BE, Blessed G, Roth M: Observations on the brains of demented old people. J Neurol Sci 11:205–242, 1970

Wechsler D: A standardized memory scale for clinical use. J Psychol 19:87–95, 1945

3

Familial Alzheimer's Disease

Marshall Folstein, M.D.
John C. S. Breitner, M.D.
Diane Powell, M.D.

3

Familial Alzheimer's Disease

Evidence will be reviewed from the literature and our own studies which suggests that a large segment of the cases of Alzheimer's disease seen in an outpatient clinic are transmitted as an autosomal dominant, age-dependent disorder.

Alzheimer described the clinical pathological entity that bears his name in 1907. The familial form (FAD) was recognized first in 1926 (Meggendorfer 1926). Although a genetic etiology for this condition has been hypothesized on various occasions, this hypothesis has not been adequately tested and consequently remains unrefuted. Due to aging of the population as a whole, conditions will be appropriate in the next few years to test the autosomal dominant hypothesis because families composed of a large number of elderly relatives will facilitate family studies and linkage studies. Such studies depend on an accurate phenotype (Folstein and Powell, in press; Breitner and Folstein, in press).

The Alzheimer's disease phenotype is a clinical pathological entity. The clinical symptoms have been reported in the literature since 1837 when Prichard described an entity he called "senile incoherence," which progressed from impaired memory to loss of reasoning to incomprehension and loss of instinctive action (Prichard 1837). The clinical features of Alzheimer's patient indicated the presence of amnesia, aphasia, and probably apraxia (Alzheimer

1907). And again, in 1952, Sjogren et al., described a case series indicating that 80 percent of individuals with the presenile (early) onset of dementia suffer from aphasia and apraxia. A case series that included a large number of autopsies was published in 1965 by Constantinidis, who documented these same clinical features in late-onset as well as early-onset cases (Constantinidis 1978). This observation was repeated by Lauter and Meyer (1968).

Because these studies included careful clinical description of symptoms and, in some cases, examination of neuropathological material, we conclude that the clinical course of the syndrome associated with Alzheimer's neuropathology beginning either before or after the age of 65 years classically presents as amnesia followed by aphasia and apraxia. In these series, the severity of symptoms increased steadily, with death occurring after eight to ten years of illness.

Studies by Blessed et al. (1968), and later by Perry et al. (1978), clearly indicate that the severity of the clinical symptoms is correlated with the severity of neuropathological changes—either the senile plaques or, in Perry's report, the cholinesterase deficiency. Appropriate studies have not been conducted in which clinicians and neuropathologists, each blind to the diagnosis of the other, arrived at independent diagnoses so that specificity and sensitivity of a given set of diagnostic criteria could be estimated. Our own work indicates that strict criteria predict 80 to 90 percent of cases on autopsy. We conclude that clinical symptoms, as they develop through several years of illness, are valid indicators of a clinical pathological entity. But are these symptoms a predictor of those cases with a genetic etiology?

HEREDITARY TRANSMISSION

To investigate the hereditary transmission of Alzheimer's disease, two types of family studies have been conducted: population studies and extended pedigree studies. The population studies of Alzheimer's disease indicate that the disorder is found in particular families more often than in the general population (Meggendorfer 1926; Sjogren et al. 1952; Constantinidis 1978; Larsson 1963;

Akesson 1969; Heston et al. 1966; Heston 1978; Heston et al. 1981; Breitner and Folstein, in press). From these studies we can conclude that the first-degree relatives of a patient with Alzheimer's disease has three to four times the risk of developing this disorder as the general population. However, the various investigators have not found that the cases are distributed within families in a particular Mendelian pattern such as dominant, recessive, or sex-linked.

There have been more than 50 extended pedigree reports of FAD (Cook et al. 1979). The details published with two of these reports enabled us to determine that the patients were suffering from classical Alzheimer's disease. The pedigree reported by Lauter (1961), in which 13 members were affected in five generations and in which three cases were pathologically proven (including a concordant twin-pair), is a clear example. The pedigree reported by Feldman et al. (1963) is another. The typical age of onset in both of these pedigrees was well below the age of 65 years. In these pedigrees the classical course of amnesia followed by aphasia and apraxia predicted the neuropathology and predicted familial disorder suggesting autosomal dominant distribution.

PRESENT STUDY

Our own work in this area suggests that the classical course of an insidious onset of amnesia followed in several years by prominent aphasia and apraxia when applied to cases, without risk factors for vascular disease such as hypertension and diabetes, predicts a lifetime risk to relatives near 50 percent, if appropriate means of analysis take into account the censoring effect of individuals dying before they become at risk for the disease (Folstein and Breitner 1981; Breitner and Folstein, in press). Expression of the disease appears strongly age-dependent, but 50 percent lifetime incidence is the proportion that would be expected in an autosomal dominant (but age-dependent) disorder.

These results were obtained by studying the relatives of a population of patients found in nursing homes. If, in nursing homes, Alzheimer's disease cases were ascertained according to strict diagnostic criteria from history and chart review, then two groups of demented individuals could be found. One group was demented, with symptoms of aphasia and agraphia shown directly by inability to write a spontaneous sentence—agraphic cases. The average age of this group was 82 years and they had 192 relatives over 55 years of age who were at risk. Another group of 14 *nonagraphic*, demented probands (mean age, 85 years) had 70 relatives at risk. Both groups of patients were ill for approximately seven years. The patients who met criteria for a dementia syndrome (excluding vascular disease) progressing in the classical way—with a prominent agraphia—had more relatives who became demented than did the demented individuals of similar age and duration of illness without agraphia. Thirty-three age- and sex-matched, nondemented controls in the same nursing homes had 157 relatives at risk. Of these, only 3 percent were demented compared to 11 percent of relatives for the agraphic group.

When appropriate survival analysis was applied to these data, we found that the sibs and children of agraphic probands had 55.7 percent lifetime risk, while parents, sibs, and children combined had a 44 percent lifetime risk. Those who were demented but did not have the classical symptoms of Alzheimer's disease showed no increased risk of dementia in their relatives, compared with controls. When the various survival curves were plotted they showed that our data were similar to data reported by others (Heston et al. 1981; Larsson 1969) for the early stages of the illness, but that the rates were higher at 90 years of age in the current series. We attributed this difference to the selection criteria of the patients.

The different proportions of affected family members suggest that there are at least two types of dementia syndrome previously attributed clinically to Alzheimer's disease. One type—with classical symptoms—shows a strong familial aggregation, while the other type—without the classical symptoms—seems to appear in this population sporadically.

In a second study, conducted in our clinic, we studied the prevalence and ages of onset of all familial cases meeting classical criteria, ascertained over a three-year period.

PREVALENCE

The prevalence of FAD is unknown. The determination of prevalence is hindered by the necessity for developing extensive pedigrees on individuals with diseases extending back many decades and generations, and the need to limit the survey to those families in which individual members lived long enough to express the disease. However, even if crude counts are taken, a substantial number of cases presenting to a clinic are familial. The exact proportion will depend on the diagnostic criteria and the extent of the genealogical effort devoted to the pedigrees. Our own data suggest that one might expect more than half of all Alzheimer's disease cases to be familial.

ANALYSIS

Analysis of the 21 clinic pedigrees by age of onset indicated that the age of onset of familial cases is from 27 to 81 years. There was a correlation between the age of onset of dementia in the proband and in the affected relatives (Powell and Folstein, in press). Thus cases with a very early age of onset tended also to have very early onset in affected family members, while cases with a late age of onset tended also to have late onset in the family. There were, of course, many families in which there was a wide range of ages of onset within the family. The "breeding true" in the age of onset within families is a demonstration of phenotypic heterogeneity, and suggests the possibility of genetic heterogeneity. Thus, in Alzheimer's disease there are probably two types of heterogeneity: (1) familial versus nonfamilial cases and (2) among familial cases, possibly several specific disorders, which are suggested by their differing ages of onset.

A further analysis of the clinic pedigrees suggested that many of the families have transmission over three generations and that there is no statistically greater number of females than males, both of which are compatible with an autosomal dominant mode of transmission of age-dependent onset.

That clear examples of multigenerational pedigrees have been found and are not rare would invite linkage experiments with the new recombinant DNA technology. Only after a marker for the Alzheimer's gene has been found and its distribution studied within families will the hypothesis that Alzheimer's disease is an autosomal dominant with age-dependent expression be tested.

SUMMARY

Numerous studies find that Alzheimer's disease is familial, and pedigrees have been reported in which Alzheimer's disease appears to be transmitted as an age-dependent autosomal dominant trait. The classical symptoms predict the familial type, which occurs in more than half of all pedigrees researched in an outpatient dementia clinic.

References

Akesson HO: A population study of senile and arteriosclerotic psychoses. Hum Hered 19:546–566, 1969

Alzheimer A: Über eine eigenartige Erkrankung der Hirnrinde. Allgemeine Zeitschrift für Psychiatrie und Psychisch-Gerichtliche Medizin 64:146–148, 1907

Blessed G, Tomlinson BE, Roth M: The association between quantitative measures of dementia and of senile changes in the cerebral grey matter of elderly subjects. Br J Psychiatr 114:797–811, 1968

Breitner JCS, Folstein MF: Familial Alzheimer's dementia: a prevalent disorder with specific clinical features. Psychol Med (in press)

Constantinidis J: Is Alzheimer's disease a major form of senile dementia? Clinical, anatomical, and genetic data, in Alzheimer's Disease: Senile Dementia and Related Disorders. Edited by Katzman R, Terry RD, Bick KL. New York, Raven Press, 1978

Cook RH, Ward BE, Austin JH: Studies in aging of the brain, IV: familial Alzheimer's disease: relation to transmissible dementia, aneuploidy, and microtubular defects. Neurology 29:1402–1412, 1979

Feldman RG, Chandler KA, Levy LL, et al: Familial Alzheimer's disease. Neurology 13:811–824, 1963

Folstein MF, Breitner JCS: Language disorder predicts familial Alzheimer's disease. Johns Hopkins Med J 149:145–147, 1981

Folstein MF, Powell D: Is Alzheimer's disease inherited? A methodological review. Integrative Psychiatry (in press)

Heston LL: Pedigrees of thirty families with Alzheimer's disease: associations with defective organization of microfilaments and microtubulas. Behav Genet 8:315–331, 1978

Heston LL, Louther DLW, Levanthal CM: Alzheimer's disease: a family study. Arch Neurol 15:225–233, 1966

Heston LL, Mastri AR, Anderson E, et al: Dementia of the Alzheimer type: clinical genetics, natural history, and associated conditions. Arch Gen Psychiatry 38:1085–1090, 1981

Larsson T, Sjogren T, Jacobsen G: Senile dementia. Acta Psychiatr Scand [Suppl] 39:1–259, 1963

Lauter H: Genealogische Erhebungen in einer familie mit Alzheimerscher Krankheit. Arch Psychiat Nervenkr 202:126, 1961

Lauter H, Meyer JE: Clinical and nosological concepts of senile dementia, in Senile Dementia. Edited by Muller C, Compi L. Bern, Hans Huber, 1968

Meggendorfer F: Über die hereditäre Disposition zu Dementia Senilis. Z Neurol Psychiatry 101:387–405, 1926

Perry EK, Tomlinson BE, Blessed G, et al: Correlation of cholinergic abnormalities with senile plaques and mental test scores in senile dementia. Br Med J 2:1457–1459, 1978

Powell D, Folstein MF: Pedigree study of familial Alzheimer's disease. Journal of Neurogenetics (in press)

Prichard JC: A Treatise on Insanity and Other Disorders Affecting the Mind. Philadelphia, Haswell, Barnington & Haswell, 1837, pp 69–80

Sjogren T, Sjogren H, Lindgren AGH: Morbus Alzheimer and morbus Pick: genetic, clinical, and patho-anatomical study. Acta Psychiatrica et Neurologica Scandinavica. Supplement. 82:1–152, 1952

4

The Philothermal Response and the Diagnosis of Dementia of the Alzheimer's Type

Steven S. Matsuyama, Ph.D.
Tsu-ker Fu, Ph.D.
John O. Kessler, Ph.D.
Lissy F. Jarvik, M.D., Ph.D.

4

The Philothermal Response and the Diagnosis of Dementia of the Alzheimer's Type

The clinical diagnosis of dementia of the Alzheimer's type (DAT) is most difficult to make and remains a challenge. At the moment, short of a biopsy or postmortem neuropathological examination, there is no clinical laboratory test or combination of tests specific to DAT that can positively confirm the diagnosis. Thus, DAT is a diagnosis of exclusion requiring an extensive battery of screening tests such as is recommended by the Task Force sponsored by the National Institute on Aging (1980). Compared to the availability of a positive diagnostic marker, this approach is not cost effective. Consequently, there is an ongoing search for biological markers to aid in the diagnosis. Examples include immunocytochemistry of paired helical filaments (Ihara et al. 1983), fibroblast phosphofructokinase activity (Sorbi and Blass 1983), erythrocyte lithium countertransport rates (Diamond et al. 1983), and the cellular philothermal response presented in detail below. Since DAT most likely represents a disorder of heterogeneous etiology and a given biological marker may identify only one homogeneous subgroup of patients, several markers may emerge. It is hoped that these potential markers may shed light on the etiology and pathogenesis of DAT and lead to rational treatment and ultimately to preventive measures.

METHODS

An area of specific research interest to us has been the evaluation of the tendency for cellular migration along a temperature gradient toward the higher temperature, which we have designated as the philothermal response (*philo*, having a strong attraction to or affinity for, and *therm*, heat). The experimental procedure to quantitate the philothermal response was developed in our laboratory (Kessler et al. 1979; Fu et al. 1982), and its design allows the application of a temperature gradient while avoiding the forces of thermal convection. In brief, the basic methodology is as follows: A sample of venous blood is drawn, and a polymorphonuclear leukocyte (PMN) cell suspension is prepared by a two-step Ficoll-Hypaque density centrifugation and dextran sedimentation. This cell suspension is then added to hollow, flat, glass microslides that were previously partially filled with an agarose gel (0.75 pcrcent) solution. The prepared microslides are then exposed to a temperature gradient (1.4 C/mm) for three hours. Sequential observation of the philothermal response at hourly intervals reveals an increasing number of cells that have migrated from the cell suspension source toward the warmer temperature at the agarose-glass interface. In routine evaluations, photomicrographs are taken after three hours, and the response is quantitated from these photographic enlargements. Each photograph is analyzed independently by at least two observers, and only upon completion of the analysis is the code broken. Quantitation includes the total number of responding cells as well as their spatial distribution.

Philothermal locomotion is a function of the magnitude of the temperature gradient and the cell concentration. To assess the stability of the method, the philothermal response of PMNs from two nominally healthy volunteers was examined over an interval of 55 days. Repeat determinations revealed considerable day-to-day variability, but there was no overlap in response measures between the two volunteers (Fu et al. 1982).

Our initial investigation addressed the philothermal response in relation to aging since with advancing age there is a slight lowering of normal body temperature and often a reduced febrile response to infection. No age-related changes were detected in nominally healthy volunteers. Theoretically, an abnormal loco-motory response may be expected in patients with DAT for several reasons. (1) Microtubules are important in cell orientation and directed cell migration (Malech et al. 1977), and Heston (1976) has postulated a microtubular defect in DAT. (2) Microtubules play an essential role in chromosome separations, and a microtu-bular basis has been postulated for the increased frequency of aneuploidy reported in individuals with DAT (Matsuyama, in press). (3) An increased frequency of individuals with Down's syndrome has been reported among DAT families (Heston, 1976). Down's syndrome, which is primarily the result of a trisomic condition (trisomy 21), is accompanied by the neurofibrillary tangles and senile plaques characteristic of DAT (Jervis 1948; Burger and Vogel 1973) in patients who survive long enough to reach at least the fifth decade of life. (4) Defective cell migration has been reported in Down's syndrome patients (Khan et al. 1975) as well as in other individuals with chromosomal abnormalities (Seger et al. 1976). (5) The philothermal response may represent another host defense mechanism, distinct from chemotaxis, that is directed at inflammation and infection. Patients with DAT often have poor resistance to infection, and this poor resistance may be the result of a compromised host defense system. Thus, on the basis of the above theoretical arguments, we examined the philothermal response of PMNs obtained from patients with a clinical diagnosis of DAT (Jarvik et al. 1982).

RESULTS AND DISCUSSION

We evaluated 18 patients with DAT, 10 men and eight women, ranging in age from 55 to 90 years with a mean ± SD age of 74 ± 10.2 years. The clinical diagnosis was made in accordance with the DSM-III criteria for primary degenerative dementia following a psychiatric interview, neurological examination, and routine clin-ical laboratory tests (including thyroid function and serology). Computed tomography scans available for 15 (83 percent) and electroencephalograms for 13 (72 percent) were consistent with a diagnosis of DAT. Our comparison group included 18 relatively healthy individuals without mental disorder matched by sex and age as best as we could to the DAT patients. These 10 men and eight women ranged in age from 57 to 89 years with a mean $\pm$ SD age of 72.9 $\pm$ 7.6 years.

Several measures were used to quantify the philothermal response. Initially we compared the total number of migrating cells (N) for the DAT patients, the mean $\pm$ SD was 271 $\pm$ 140 (range 88–555). The comparison individuals without mental disorder had a mean of 258 $\pm$ 97 (range 89–436). The difference in mean numbers of migrating cells was not statistically significant. However, we did find a significant difference between group means for the leading front measure (the distance migrated by the five cells farthest from the cell suspension source). In the DAT patients the mean $\pm$ SD was 808 $\pm$ 160 μm, ranging from 439 to 1122 μm; for the comparison group, the mean was 98 $\pm$ 126 μm, with a range from 725 to 1171 μm. Thus, although the total number was not significantly different, the leading front measure indicated a difference in the spatial distribution of the responding cell population.

In light of this finding, we sought another statistical parameter of the philothermal response applicable to each individual's cellular response that might discriminate patients from controls. This parameter, the value R, may be the most meaningful clinically and represents the ratio of the number of proximal cells (cells in the interval 210–420 μm from the cell suspension source) to the number of distal cells (cells beyond 700 μm). Thus, a high R value is found when there are few distally migrated cells.

The individual R values for the DAT patients and comparison individuals were calculated. The number of cells in the proximal interval represented approximately 25 percent of the total number of responding cells for both DAT and comparison individuals. Of the 18 DAT patients, the R values ranged from 4.8 to infinity, and 15 (83 percent) had R values greated than 11. The 18 healthy, mentally normal individuals had a similar range of R values (4.2–12.8), but only one had an R value greater than 11. The R value as a function of the number of responding cells (N) was examined, and, overall, we did find a significant negative correlation between N and R ($r = -38$, p .05). However, the correlation between N and R was significant only for the DAT group ($r = -.53$), not for the comparison group ($r = -.19$).

It is important to determine the replicability of the R value. We have repeat determinations on seven individuals at intervals ranging from one day to two years. While we did find considerable variability, the R values, which had all been below 11 initially, remained below 11 at the second determination. The variability was not unexpected since the current method of analysis is static (quantitation from photomicrographs taken after three hours of exposure to the temperature gradient), while the philothermal response is a dynamic process.

Based on these results, the philothermal response as quantified by the R value appears to differentiate at least a subgroup of DAT patients from individuals without mental disorder. Although none of the comparison individuals have died, four of the 18 DAT patients have, all with R values greater than 11, and autopsies were performed on three of them. For each case, the neuropathological examination confirmed the clinical diagnosis.

Since the differentiation by R value does not necessarily imply diagnostic specificity, we evaluated the response of patients with multi-infarct dementia (MID) and unipolar depression. The three MID patients (one man and two women), ranging in age from 66 to 74 years, with a duration of illness from four to 10 years, all were found to have low R values (3.0, 4.2, and 4.3). The seven depressed patients (three men and four women) ranged in age from 50 to 70 years, and six of them had an R value of less than 11. The exception was a 63-year-old man with an R value of 11.2. These findings, then, suggest that the nonspecific accompaniments of dementing illness and the symptoms of depression often seen in patients with DAT are *not* responsible for the decreased numbers of distally migrated cells as quantified by R values greater than 11.

Clearly, we need to evaluate a larger sample of DAT patients, as well as patients with non-DAT dementias (e.g., MID, Huntington's disease) and physical illnesses (e.g., rheumatoid arthritis).

The impaired cell migration in DAT patients was not a function of age, sex, or duration of illness. We also examined in detail the health status and medications for each of the 36 individuals. The results indicate that for the DAT patients no single physical illness (e.g., hypertension or osteoarthritis) was associated with an elevated ratio ($R > 11$). Most of the patients were taking medications (diuretics, phenothiazines, and tricyclic antidepressants were the most common), but those who were not also had elevated R values. Many of the comparison individuals were not taking any medications, including the individuals with the high R value. We also examined the records of the three MID patients and found the following medical diagnoses: hypertension and atrial fibrillation with angina for one patient, a spinal deformation since childhood for another, and none for the third. These three patients had been taking the following medications: methyldopa, dipyridamole, digitalis, amitryptyline, doxepin, and tranquilizers (used regularly) for the first patient; multivitamins for the second; ergoloid mesylates, dipyridamole, and acetaminophen for the third. The records of the seven depressed patients showed that five had been receiving tricyclic antidepressants (four recieved imipramine and one received doxepin). The one depressed individual who had an elevated R value was receiving imipramine, as were three others with R values less than 11.

Unfortunately, we are not aware of the underlying basis of the abnormal spatial distribution reflected in the elevated R value. Is there a deficit of a fast-moving subpopulation of cells, or is it the result of less effective directed migration? And is the abnormality related to a microtubular defect? Alternatively, do the individual cells move with slower average speed, do the cells slow down over time, or is it the result of cell-cell interactions? Indeed, in-situ observations have shown numerous collisions occurring in the migration space. These questions are by no means exhaustive, and while none can be answered at this time, our studies suggest that the cellular philothermal response is compromised in a subgroup of DAT patients.

In addition to the evaluation of the philothermal response of cells obtained from DAT patients, we investigated whether or not exogenous factors present in the sera of patients are capable of modulating the philothermal response of normal cells (Matsuyama and Fu 1983). For these experiments, we assessed the effects of sera obtained from patients with a clinical diagnosis of DAT compared to sera obtained from young and elderly, healthy, mentally normal individuals on cells derived from healthy normal adults. Serum samples were obtained from four patients with DAT, two men (age, 61 and 83 years) and two women (age, 73 and 85 years) with a mean age of 75.5 years; four nominally healthy, mentally normal elderly individuals matched for age and sex to the DAT patients, two men (age, 61 and 87 years) and two women (age, 69 and 84 years) with a mean age of 75.2 years; and four healthy young adults, two men (age, 24 and 36 years) and two women (age, 28 and 33 years) with a mean age of 30.2 years.

PMNs were obtained from three healthy, nondemented individuals: one woman (age, 28 years) and two men (age, 36 and 87 years). The individual cell suspensions were aliquotted, and the serum sample to be tested was added to each aliquot. The samples were all coded and dispensed by an individual who was not directly involved in the experiments. The suspensions were then used to fill the microslide preparations, which were subsequently exposed to the temperature gradient for three hours.

The results were quite striking. In the presence of serum from normal adults, a large number of cells migrated from the cell suspension source; the response ranged from 194 to 352 cells. For the normal elderly it ranged from 137 to 217 cells. By contrast, the philothermal response of cells derived from normal adults was significantly reduced in the presence of serum obtained from DAT patients, with means of 12, 13, and 20 migrating cells. Not surprisingly, the difference between serum from DAT patients and serum from normal elderly was statistically significant ($p < .001$). Clearly, a factor, or factors, in the serum of these four DAT patients was capable of inhibiting the philothermal response. What this factor, or factors, may be remains to be explored.

We asked whether or not the sera from the Alzheimer patients acted as a chemoattractant and for that reason cells were not capable of exhibiting a "normal" philothermal response. We investigated this possibility and found only one of the four patient sera exhibited any chemoattractant activity. Thus, chemoattraction cannot explain the consistently reduced cellular response in the presence of sera from DAT patients. Therefore, the significantly reduced philothermal response of cells obtained from the three healthy volunteers in the presence of sera obtained from patients with clinically diagnosed DAT suggests that factors present in the sera are capable of modifying the response of cells to migrate along a temperature gradient.

SUMMARY

To summarize, the preliminary results of our studies indicate that the philothermal response holds promise as a positive diagnostic test for DAT. Cellular as well as humoral factors may differentiate a subgroup of DAT patients from healthy aged individuals. Since our pilot data, however, are based on but a small number of subjects, replication is clearly needed. Moreover, numerous basic parameters of the philothermal response remain to be explored.

References

Burger PC, Vogel FS: The development of the pathologic changes of Alzheimer's disease and senile dementia in patients with Down's syndrome. Am J Pathol 73:457–468, 1973

Diamond JM, Matsuyama SS, Meier K, et al: Elevation of erythrocyte countertransport rates in dementia of the Alzheimer type. N Engl J Med 309:1061–1062, 1983

Fu TK, Kessler JO, Jarvik LF, et al: Philothermal and chemotactic locomotion of leukocytes: methods and results. Cell Biophys 4:77–95, 1982

Heston LL: Alzheimer's disease, trisomy 21, and myeloproliferative disorders: associations suggesting a genetic diathesis. Science 196:322–323, 1976

Ihara Y, Abraham C, Selkoe DJ: Antibodies to paired helical filaments in Alzheimer's disease do not recognize normal brain proteins. Nature 304:727–730, 1983

Jarvik LF, Matsuyama SS, Kessler JO, et al: Philothermal response of polymorphonuclear leukocytes in dementia of the Alzheimer's type. Neurobiol Aging 3:93–99, 1982

Jervis GA: Early senile dementia in mongoloid idiocy. Am J Psychiatry 105:102–106, 1948

Kessler JO, Jarvik LF, Fu TK, et al: Thermotaxis, chemotaxis and age. Age 2:5–11, 1979

Khan AJ, Evans HE, Glass L, et al: Defective neutrophil chemotaxis in patients with Down's syndrome. J Pediatr 87:87–89, 1975

Malech HL, Root RK, Gallin JI: Structural analysis of human neutrophil migration: centriole, microtubule, and microfilament orientation and function during chemotaxis. J Cell Biol 75:666–693, 1977

Matsuyama SS: Genetic factors in dementia of the Alzheimer's type, in Alzheimer's Disease: The Standard Reference. Edited by Reisberg B. New York, Free Press, 1983, pp 155–160

Matsuyama SS, Fu TK: Inhibition of normal polymorphonuclear philothermal response by serum from dementia of the Alzheimer's type patients. Age 6:72–75, 1983

National Institute on Aging Task Force: Senility reconsidered: treatment possibilities for mental impairment in the elderly. JAMA 233:259–263, 1980

Seger D, Wildfever A, Bushinger G, et al: Defects in granulocyte function in various chromosome abnormalities. Klin Wochenschr 54:177–183, 1976

Sorbi S, Blass JP: Fibroblast phosphofructokinase in Alzheimer disease and Down syndrome. Banbury Report 15:297–308, 1983

5

Monoamines and Monoamine Oxidase in Primary Degenerative Dementia

George S. Alexopoulos, M.D.
Kenneth W. Lieberman, Ph.D.
Robert C. Young, M.D.
Charles A. Shamoian, M.D., Ph.D.

5

Monoamines and Monoamine Oxidase in Primary Degenerative Dementia

Dementia is the major psychiatric syndrome of old age. Approximately 5 percent of the population over 65 years old have severe dementia and 12 percent have mild-to-moderate dementia (Katzman 1976; Terry 1976). Although various disorders can lead to a dementia syndrome, the majority of elderly demented patients (50 to 70 percent) suffer from primary degenerative dementia (PDD).

The etiology of PDD is unknown. After the description of "non-infarct dementia" by Alzheimer in 1899, the dominant view was that the cause of this dementia was brain arteriosclerosis. However, Corsellis and Evans (1965) and later Tomlinson et al. (1970) observed that psychiatrically normal elderly subjects had almost as many arteriosclerotic changes in their brain blood vessels as demented patients. These findings established PDD as a clinical and neuropathological entity distinct from dementias of vascular etiology. Macroscopically, patients with PDD have cortical atrophy with various degrees of ventricular dilatation, although brain weight is similar to that of age-matched normal controls. The microscopic changes in PDD include neurofibrillary tangles, senile plaques, and granulovacuolar bodies in the cortex and the hippocampus. These neuropathological changes are not etiologically specific for PDD (Schneck et al. 1982).

Multiple pathophysiological abnormalities have been reported in PDD. The best-documented abnormality is reduction of acetylcholine neurotransmission in the brain (Bartus et al. 1982). Despite these findings, cholinomimetic agents have failed to improve memory functions substantially in PDD patients. This has been attributed to the methodological complexity of these clinical studies. However, another reason may be that other neurotransmitters may be abnormal in PDD.

STUDIES OF BRAIN MONOAMINES

Originally, Gottfries et al. (1969) reported reduced levels of the dopamine metabolite homovanillic acid (HVA) in the caudate nucleus, the putamen, and the globus pallidus in patients with PDD compared to age-matched normal controls. HVA concentration in the caudate has been reported to be negatively correlated with intellectual impairment (Gottfries et al. 1969; Winblab et al. 1982). HVA concentrations in the caudate were relatively lower in PDD patients with onset of illness at 65 years or earlier, compared to patients with a later onset of illness (Winblab et al. 1982). Furthermore, PDD patients with an early age of illness onset had a stronger negative correlation between HVA levels and memory impairment (Spearman's $r = .70$) than did late-onset PDD patients (Spearman's $r = .42$), suggesting a biological difference between these two groups of patients. The concentration of HVA in the cerebrospinal fluid (CSF) has been found to be reduced in patients with PDD compared to normal control subjects (Gottfries et al. 1970). Mann et al. (1980) failed to replicate these findings. However, HVA concentrations in the CSF of PDD patients have been reported to be similar to those of nondemented patients with Parkinson's disease, which is a disorder characterized by reduced levels of dopamine and HVA in striatum and decreased levels in CSF (Growdon and Logue 1982). In autopsies, patients with PDD had reduced dopamine levels in the caudate and the hypothalamus compared to age-matched normal control subjects (Winblab et al. 1982).

Postmortem studies have demonstrated a reduction of norepinephrine in the hippocampus, the cingulate gyrus, the caudate, and the hypothalamus in patients with PDD compared to elderly normal controls (Adolfsson et al. 1978, 1979; Winblab et al. 1982). Brain norepinephrine levels were negatively correlated with intellectual impairment. However, the metabolite of norepinephrine, 3-methoxy-4-hydroxy phenylethylglycol (MHPG), has been found to be increased in the cingulate gyrus and the caudate of patients with PDD (Carlsson et al. 1979; Winblab et al. 1982). The increase of MHPG has been attributed to increased norepinephrine turnover in the brain. However, this finding was not replicated by another group (Mann et al. 1980).

Reduced concentrations of serotonin have been found in the hippocampus, the cingulate gyrus, the caudate, and the hypothalamus in PDD patients compared to age-matched normal controls (Winblab et al. 1982). PDD patients with onset of illness prior to the 65th year had lower brain serotonin than patients who developed PDD at a later age. Reduction of serotonin's metabolite 5-hydroxy-indolacetic acid (5-HIAA) has also been found in the hypothalamus and the hippocampus of patients with PDD compared to normal controls (Winblab et al. 1982). Concentrations of 5-HIAA in these brain areas were found to negatively correlate with intellectual impairment in PDD patients.

With some exceptions (Mann et al. 1980) the majority of reports suggest a reduction of brain monoamine neurotransmitter concentration in a subgroup of PDD patients. Several factors may contribute to the decline of brain monoamines in these patients, one of which may be increased activity of their catabolic enzyme monoamine oxidase (MAO).

STUDIES OF PLATELET MONOAMINE OXIDASE ACTIVITY

MAO is responsible for the catabolism of monoamines through oxidative deamination and participates in the regulation of the intraneuronal levels of these neurotransmitters (Kopin 1964; Spector et al. 1967). Platelet MAO activity has been considered to be an indirect indicator of brain MAO activity because the platelet has many similarities to the neuron (Sandler et al.1981). Furthermore, demographic variables such as age and sex influence both platelet and brain MAO activity in the same direction (Robinson and Nies 1980).

We studied platelet MAO activity in patients with primary degenerative dementia and hypothesized that this group has higher platelet MAO activity than same-age normal control subjects.

Method

The subjects were psychiatric inpatients and the control group consisted of normal volunteers, without personal or family history of psychiatric disorders, who lived in the community. None of the subjects were receiving neuroleptics, tricyclic antidepressants, MAO inhibitors, lithium carbonate, insulin, nitroglycerine, guanethidine, or L-dopa, which have been reported to influence platelet MAO activity (Robinson and Nies 1980). Diagnosis was made using DSM-III criteria by two psychiatrists. Cognitive symptoms were rated with the Mini-Mental State Examination (MMSE) (Folstein et al. 1975) and the Cognitive Capacity State Examination (CCSE) (Jacobs et al. 1977). Symptoms of depression were rated with the 24-item Hamilton Depression Rating Scale (HDRS) (Hamilton 1960). The Schedule for Affective Disorders and Schizophrenia (SADS) (Spitzer et al. 1975) was used to document and quantify other psychiatric symptoms. The course of primary degenerative dementia was defined as acute (less than six months), subacute (six months to one year), subchronic (one to five years), and chronic (more than five years), depending on the interval between the onset of illness and the development of moderate dementia (Hughes et al. 1982).

Blood was drawn between 8:00 and 10:00 A.M. in vacuum tubes containing acid dextrose citrate. After a series of centrifugations a platelet pellet was prepared and stored at -20 C up to 20 days. Platelet MAO activity was assayed using benzylamine as substrate (Bockar et al. 1974). Protein was assayed with the Lowry method (Lowry et al. 1951). Platelet MAO activity was expressed in nmol/mg protein per hour.

Student's t-test and Spearman's rank order correlation (r_s) and

Pearson's product moment correlations (r_p) were used to analyze the data. The significance levels are two tailed.

Results

Of the 51 subjects, 31 were patients with PDD without history or presence of other psychiatric disorders, and 20 were same-age

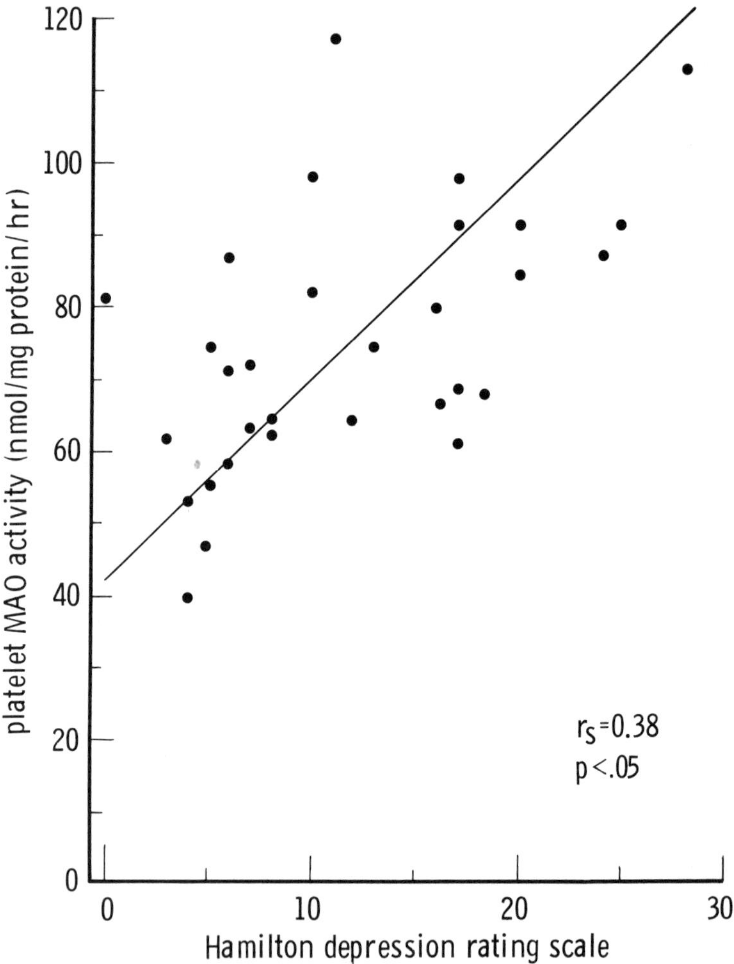

Figure 1 Platelet Monoamine Oxidase Activity Compared to Hamilton Depression Rating Scale Scores in 31 Patients with Primary Degenerative Dementia.

normal controls. There was no significant age difference between PDD patients (mean ± SD, 76.7 ± 8.1 years) and normal control subjects (73.6 ± 4.8). Platelet MAO activity was significantly higher in 31 patients with primary degenerative dementia (mean ± SD MAO activity, 74.6 ± 18.0) than in 20 normal control subjects (61.5 ± 19.2) ($t = 2.79$, $df = 49$, $p < .05$). The sex of subjects has been reported to influence platelet MAO activity (Robinson and Nies 1980). For this reason platelet MAO activity of women was analyzed separately. Women with PDD ($N = 25$; mean ± SD MAO activity, 78.0 ± 16.1) had significantly higher platelet MAO activity than female control subjects ($N = 16$; 66.0 ± 18.5) ($t = 2.49$, $df = 39$, $p < .05$).

Platelet MAO activity had a significant positive correlation with age in elderly normal subjects ($r = .51$, $df = 18$, $p < .05$). However, platelet MAO activity did not correlate with age in patients with PDD ($r_p = .03$).

The effect of psychiatric symptoms on platelet MAO activity of patients with PDD was examined. Platelet MAO activity had a positive correlation with HDRS scores ($r_s = .38$, $p < .05$) (Figure 1). Patients with delusions ($N = 10$; mean ± SD MAO activity, 73.7 ± 16.3) had indistinguishable platelet MAO activity from demented patients without delusions ($N = 21$; 75.0 ± 19.2). Demented patients with hallucinations ($N = 4$; 82.9 ± 20.7) had comparable values with nonhallucinating patients ($N = 27$; 73.4 ± 17.7). Presence of anxiety did not influence platelet MAO activity in patients with PDD. Patients without anxiety ($N = 16$; 69.8 ± 16.9) had similar platelet MAO activity to that of demented patients with mild anxiety (SADS psychic anxiety, 2–3) ($N = 9$; 81.4 ± 18) or severe anxiety (SADS psychic anxiety, 4–6) ($N = 6$, 77.7 ± 21.1) ($F_{2-28} = 1.3$, $p > .05$).

There was a significant positive correlation between platelet MAO activity and chronicity of PDD (Figure 2).

Comment

In this sample of patients with PDD, platelet monoamine oxidase was significantly higher than in normal elderly controls. Our findings are in agreement with those of Adolfsson et al.

(1980). They observed an elevation of platelet and brain MAO activity in a smaller group of patients with PDD, using different substrates for the MAO assay. The increase of MAO activity in both platelet and the brain of patients with PDD suggests that this

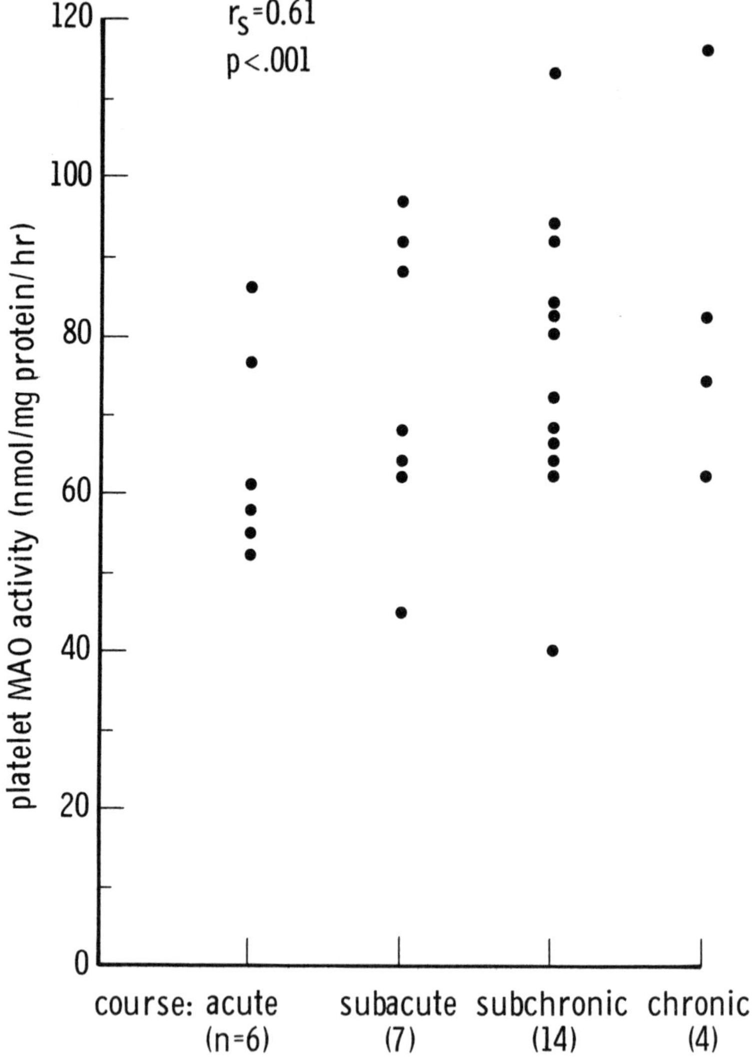

Figure 2 Platelet Monoamine Oxidase Activity Compared to Chronicity in 31 Patients with Primary Degenerative Dementia.

disorder leads to a widespread disturbance of the MAO system.

A significant correlation between age and platelet MAO activity was found in the group of elderly normal control subjects. However, age did not correlate with platelet MAO activity in patients with PDD. It appears that the disease or other factors interfere with the aging process of the platelet MAO system.

In this sample of demented patients, HDRS (mean ± SD, 11.7 ± 7) was comparable to that reported in patients with organic brain disorder (16.7 ± 8.2) (Miller 1980). Miller has reported that HDRS in organically impaired subjects correlates significantly with depression scores on Beck's Depression Inventory (0.69) and the Adjective Mood Checklist (0.75), which are both self-rating instruments. The significant correlation between HDRS and platelet MAO observed in this sample of patients suggests that elevation of platelet MAO activity may be associated with predisposition to depression in patients with PDD. However, the HDRS was constructed originally for the quantitation of symptoms of depressed patients (Hamilton 1960), and this finding therefore has to be interpreted with caution.

We observed a significant correlation between chronicity of PDD and platelet MAO activity. This finding cannot be attributed to age differences between patients with different course of illness, because age did not correlate with platelet MAO activity in subjects with PDD. PDD with a chronic course may be caused by an exaggeration of the aging process, while the more acute forms of the disease may have a different pathogenesis.

Aging leads to a decrease of brain monoamine neurotransmitters (Adolfsson et al. 1978), and a more pronounced decline of these substances has been observed in PDD (Gottfries et al. 1969; Adolfsson et al. 1978; Winblab et al. 1982). The relationship between monoamine concentrations and monoamine oxidase activity is yet to be clarified. However, in PDD changes both in brain monoamines and brain and platelet MAO activity are in the same direction with changes induced by aging. These findings suggest that an exaggeration of the aging process in these monoamine systems may predispose individuals to PDD.

CONCLUSION

Although disturbances of the cholinergic system in patients with PDD have been widely investigated, relatively little attention has been paid to changes in monoamine neurotransmission in this disorder. Recently, a reduction of monoamine neurotransmitters and an increase of their catabolic enzyme MAO has been reported in several brain areas of patients with PDD (Gottfries et al. 1969; Adolfsson et al. 1978; Winblab et al. 1982). We observed a significant ($p < .05$) increase in platelet MAO activity in patients with PDD ($N = 31$) compared to same-age controls ($N = 20$). Since changes in brain monoamines and in brain and platelet MAO activity in PDD follow the direction of changes occurring with aging, it may be that an exaggeration of such age-induced processes may predispose to this disorder. In patients with PDD there was a significant correlation between platelet MAO activity and chronicity of illness ($r = .61$), as well as with presence of depressive symptomatology ($r = .38$). These findings suggest that platelet MAO activity may distinguish subgroups of demented patients with different clinical and biochemical abnormalities and contribute to the understanding of the pathogenesis of this disorder.

References

Adolfsson R, Gottfries CG, Oreland L, et al: Reduced levels of catecholamines in the brain and increased activity of monoamine oxidase in platelets in Alzheimer's disease, in Therapeutic Implications in Alzheimer's Disease. Edited by Katzman R, Terry RD, Bick KL. New York, Raven Press, 1978

Adolfsson R, Gottfries CG, Roos BE, et al: Changes in the brain catecholamines in patients with dementia of Alzheimer's type. Br J Psychiatry 135:216–223, 1979

Adolfsson R, Gottfries CG, Oreland L, et al: Increased activity of brain and platelet monoamine oxidase in dementia of Alzheimer's type. Life Sci 27:1029–1034, 1980

Bartus RT, Dean RL, Beer B, et al: The cholinergic hypothesis of geriatric memory dysfunction. Science 217:408–417, 1982

Bockar J, Roth R, Heninger G: Increased human platelet monoamine oxidase during lithium carbonate therapy. Life Sci 15:2109–2118, 1974

Carlsson A, Adolfsson R, Aquilonius SM, et al: Biogenic amines in human brain in normal aging, senile dementia and chronic alcoholism, in Ergot Compounds and Brain Function: Neuroendocrine and Neuropsychiatric Aspects. Edited by Goldstein M. New York, Raven Press, 1979

Corsellis JAN, Evans PH: The relation of stenosis of the extracranial cerebral arteries to mental disorder and cerebral degeneration of old age, in Proceedings of the Fifth International Congress of Neuropathology. The Hague, Mouton and Co, 1965

Folstein MF, Folstein SE, McHugh PR: The Mini-Mental State. J Psychiatr Res 12:189–198, 1975

Gottfries CG, Gottfries I, Roos BE: The investigation of homovanillic acid in the human brain and its correlation to senile dementia. Br J Psychiatry 155:563–574, 1969

Gottfries CG, Gottfries I, Roos BE: Homovanillic acid and 5-hydroxyindolacetic acid in cerebrospinal fluid related to rated mental and motor impairment in senile and presenile dementia. Acta Psychiatr Scand 46:99–105, 1970

Growdon JH, Logue M: Choline and 5-HIAA levels in cerebrospinal fluid of patients with Alzheimer's disease, in Alzheimer's Disease: A Report of Progress in Research. Edited by Corkin S, Davis KL, Growdon JH, et al. New York, Raven Press, 1982, pp 35–43

Hamilton M: A psychiatric rating scale for depression (NIMH version). J Neurol Neurosurg Psychiatry 23:56–62, 1960

Hughes CP, Berg L, Danziger WL, et al: A new clinical scale for the staging of dementia. Br J Psychiatry 140:566–572, 1982

Jacobs JW, Bernhardt MR, Delgado A, et al: Screening for organic mental syndromes in mentally ill. Ann Intern Med 86:40–46, 1977

Katzman R: The prevalence and malignancy of Alzheimer's disease: a major killer. Arch Neurol 33:217–218, 1976

Kopin IJ: Storage and metabolism of catecholamines: the role of monoamine oxidase. Pharmacol Rev 16:179–191, 1964

Lowry OH, Rosebrough NH, Farr AL, et al: Protein measurement with the Folin phenol reagent. J Biol Chem 193:265–275, 1951

Mann JJ, Stanley M, Neophytides A, et al: Central amine metabolism in Alzheimer's disease: in vivo relationship to cognitive deficit. Neurobiol Aging 1:69–79, 1980

Miller NE: The measurement of mood in senile brain disease: examiner ratings and self-reports, in Psychopathology of Aging. Edited by Cole JO, Barrett JE. New York, Raven Press, 1980

Robinson DS, Nies a: Demographic, biologic and other variables affecting monoamine oxidase activity. Schizophrenia Bulletin 6:298–307, 1980

Sandler M, Reveley MA, Glover V: Human platelet monoamine oxidase activity in health and disease: a review. J Clin Pathol 34:292–302, 1981

Schneck MK, Reisberg R, Ferris SH: An overview of current concepts of Alzheimer's disease. Am J Psychiatry 139:165–173, 1982

Spector S, Gordon R, Sjoerdsma A, et al: End product inhibition of tyrosine hydroxylase as a possible mechanism for regulation of norepinephrine synthesis. Mol Pharmacol 3:549–555, 1967

Spitzer R, Endicott J, Robins E: Schedule for affective disorders and schizophrenia (SADS). New York, New York State Psychiatric Institute, 1975

Terry RD: Dementia: a brief and selective review. Arch Neurol 33:1–4, 1976

Tomlinson BE, Blessed G, Roth M: Observations on the brains of demented old people. J Neurol Sci 11:205–242, 1970.

Winblab B, Adolfsson R, Carlsson A, et al: Biogenic amines in brains of patients with Alzheimer's disease, in Alzheimer's Disease: A Report of Progress in Research. Edited by Corkin S, Davis KL, Growdon JH, et al. New York, Raven Press, 1982

6

Clinical Geriatric Psychopharmacology and Neuropeptides

Jared R. Tinklenberg, M.D.
Joe E. Thornton, M.D.
Jerome A. Yesavage, M.D.

6

Clinical Geriatric Psychopharmacology and Neuropeptides

NEUROPEPTIDES IN GERIATRIC PSYCHOPHARMACOLOGY

Neuropeptides are commonly defined as peptides produced by and active in the central nervous system. These peptides often have the same structure as peripheral hormones but can function as neurotransmitters, neuromodulators, or neurohormones (Barchas et al. 1978; Krieger and Martin 1981). Neuropeptides related to adrenocorticotropic hormone (ACTH) and those similar to vasopressin (VP) have improved animal performance in a variety of experimental paradigms, thus encouraging similar trials in humans. We will review these initial clinical studies as well as animal findings that have particular implications for the psychopharmacology of aging and dementia.

Adrenocorticotropic Hormone Peptides

Neuropeptides related to ACTH have behavioral effects that are not mediated by the pituitary or adrenals. Considerable data suggest that amino acids 4–10 (ACTH 4–10) on the 39-amino-acid ACTH molecule are responsible for most of its behavioral activity (Bohus and De Wied 1981; Rigter and Van Riezen 1979; Sandman and Kastin 1977). Since this short amino acid sequence is also shared by melanocyte-stimulating hormone (MSH), some authors name this fragment ACTH/MSH. Some studies indicate that peptide fragments as short as ACTH 4–9 or even ACTH 4–7 have behavioral activity (Witter et al. 1981). Some preclinical studies suggest that different ACTH fragments and their analogs may have multiple, independent, behavioral actions (Kastin et al. 1981). However, at the clinical level we are more impressed by their behavioral similarities, and thus we will be using the collective term ACTH-like peptides.

Many of the neurochemical effects of the ACTH-like peptides are mediated by direct brain activity rather than through peripheral mechanisms (for reviews, see Dunn and Gispen 1977; Versteeg 1980; Rigter, in press). These peptides can enhance the performance of laboratory animals on a number of experimental tasks, such as active and passive avoidance learning and maze learning, and can also enhance the restoration of performance impaired by amnestic agents (Rigter and Van Riezen 1979; Rigter, in press). Since peptides can improve performance on both positively and negatively motivated tasks, it is unlikely that they act by simply influencing sensory processes such as pain thresholds.

Although many first thought that ACTH effects were on memory per se, this now appears unlikely. Although ACTH-treated rats mastered learning reversal tasks more rapidly than did placebo-treated animals (Sandman et al. 1973), if memory alone were affected by the peptide, erroneous persevertions would be expected. Furthermore, if ACTH-like peptides improved any intrinsic aspect of memory, one would expect that all subsequent measures of that memory trace would show improvement, but this is not the case (Bohus et al. 1973). Instead, most results suggest that their effects were limited to the time period proximal to their administration; ACTH-like peptides differ from vasopressin peptides in their lack of persistent effects. In our opinion, the preclinical ACTH studies suggest that these peptides affect extrinsic memory-modulating processes that do not in themselves contain or convey information, but do influence intrinsic memory mechanisms. These modulating processes are variously described as certain kinds of arousal, attention, motivation, or mood (Pigache and Rigter 1981).

Although the first clinical trials used MSH, most recent human studies have used the ACTH peptides ACTH 4–10 or Org 2766. In animal studies both of these peptides share the behavioral properties of ACTH without stimulating the adrenal cortex to release corticosteroids. MSH/ACTH 4–10 and Org 2766 have been studied in young, cognitively unimpaired subjects and in patients with various memory deficits (Berger and Tinklenberg 1981; Pigache and Rigter 1981; Pigache, in press[a], in press[b]). The general conclusion from these studies is that no consistent effect on memory task performance was found when single-dose or short-term administration schedules were used. Occasional positive results have not been replicated convincingly. This absence of significant effects on memory has been observed in a wide variety of subjects: healthy young subjects, patients treated with electroconvulsive treatment (ECT), children with minimal brain dysfunction, alcoholics, and older people showing signs of cognitive deficit. In addition, we have been unsuccessful in attempts to specifically replicate in humans the apparent positive attentional effects of single doses of ACTH-like peptide in animals (Hunt and Tinklenberg, manuscript submitted for publication). Possible reasons for the discrepancies between animal and human responses to peptides are discussed below.

It is important to note that initial clinical trials with ACTH peptides used either single doses or relatively short periods of administration (Abuzzahab et al. 1978; Ferris et al. 1976; Branconnier et al. 1979; Dornbush et al. 1981). Short schedules of administration are, of course, appropriate in the initial stages of clinical drug development, but they produce misleading negative results with drugs that require prolonged administration before they exert significant behavior effects. It is significant that more recent studies using subchronic Org 2766 treatment schedules have been more promising. Four different investigators using subchronic, double-blind, placebo-controlled crossover designs have found positive effects of Org 2766 on depression, anxiety, and sociability in elderly patients (Ferris and Gershon 1979; Pigache, in press[a], in press[b]; Pigache and Rigter 1981). These positive results were quite consistent when treatment periods were one week or longer.

These findings suggest that ACTH peptides, especially if given in repeated-administration schedules, can enhance human performance in certain conditions. The mechanisms of action of these peptides are unclear, although as noted by Pigache (in press[c]), their positive effects on mood and sociability in certain elderly patients are clinically similar to the effects of ergoloid mesylates, the various piracetam analogs, and other "geriatric drugs." These findings suggest nonspecific actions.

Vasopressin Peptides

Normal animals treated with VP peptides show improved performance in a range of experimental tasks such as shuttle-box active and passive avoidance conditioning, pole-jumping active avoidance learning, sexually motivated maze learning, food-reinforced maze learning, reversal learning, and retrograde amnesia induced by electroconvulsive seizures, carbon dioxide, diethyldithiocarbamate, pentylenetetrazole, and puromycin treatment (Asin 1980; Bohus 1977; Bootin and Pfeiffer 1977; De Wied 1974; Hostetter et al. 1977; Rigter et al. 1974; Rigter et al. 1975). In addition, impaired performance on learning and memory tasks has been demonstrated in animals with three different conditions of VP deficiency: neurohypophysectomy, Brattleboro-type hereditary defects in the production of VP, and VP antisera treatment (De Wied 1969; De Wied et al. 1975; van Wimersma Greidanus et al. 1975). In each condition the behavioral impairment can be reversed by appropriate VP treatment. These findings indicate that VP peptides affect animal behavior through mechanisms other than simply increasing general psychomotor activity or altering sensory thresholds. Effects on memory modulating processes are more likely, and hence these peptides become of interest for clinical trials.

Other characteristics of VP peptides make them attractive for geriatric studies. Some VP analogs, such as desglycinamide arginine VP (DGAVP; Org 5667), induce the behavioral effects of the parent peptide, but without affecting cardiovascular or endocrine activity (De Wied 1980). Peptides without pressor, antidiuretic, or corticotropic effects are obviously better candidates for use in older people. Also of potential importance is that certain VP peptides exert effects on animal behavior for a few days to weeks depending on the dosage and schedule of administration (De Wied 1971). This is a longer duration of action than the ACTH-like peptides and longer than many currently available drugs with cognitive effects (e.g., most cholinergic agonists). In addition, VP peptides appear to facilitate the learning process at more than one point during the age of the memory. VP can exert positive effects on initial acquisition, immediately after acquisition when consolidation is presumably taking place, and during the subsequent retention phase when the strength of the memory trace is declining (Bohus et al. 1973; Cooper et al. 1980; De Wied 1971). This characteristic of VP peptides is also different from many other drugs that alter cognitive processes.

Two of the first clinical trials with VP in patients with cognitive impairments were positive (LeBoeuf et al. 1978; Oliveros et al. 1978), but assessments were not systematic and appropriate controls were lacking. In the first controlled study, 23 men between the ages of 50 and 65 years, who were hospitalized for minor pulmonary or gastrointestinal disorders but not screened for cognitive deficits, were randomly assigned to either lysine VP (LVP) or placebo treatment. The 12 patients who received 16 IU of LVP per day for three days performed better on attention and memory tasks (Legros et al. 1978). However, the lack of extensive baseline cognitive assessments makes it difficult to determine how comparable the two groups were before treatment and hence how much of the post-treatment scores are attributable to VP effects.

A group of investigators at the National Institute of Mental Health (NIMH) have reported a series of positive clinical trials with 1-desamino-8-D-arginine VP (DDAVP; desmopressin) (Gold et al. 1979; Weingartner et al. 1981a; Weingartner et al. 1981b). DDAVP is a VP peptide that retains antidiuretic activity but has the advantage of a longer duration of action and fewer cardiovascular effects than lysine VP or arginine VP, the naturally occurring VP peptide in humans. In the first NIMH study, four women, between the ages of 41 and 52 years, who had endogenous mood disturbances and cognitive impairment, were treated with 60–160 μg of DDAVP intranasally in a double-blind, placebo-DDAVP-placebo protocol. Three of the four patients demonstrated significant improvement in verbal learning during the three to seven weeks of DDAVP treatment. Their performance returned to baseline levels by six weeks after the end of active treatment. Two of these three cognitive responders showed some DDAVP-related mood elevation. Although the authors made rigorous attempts to maintain the double-blind, this is difficult in an A-B-A study design, especially with a substance such as DDAVP, which has antidiuretic action. In the second NIMH study, six young, cognitively unimpaired subjects demonstrated significant increases in learning and memory performance when given DDAVP intranasally for two to three weeks (Weingartner et al. 1981a). A comparison group showed no improvement. In addition, two depressed patients being treated with ECT were given either placebo or DDAVP for three days prior to ECT. Pretreatment with DDAVP reduced the characteristic retrograde amnesia that follows ECT, while placebo had no effect. In the third study, seven subjects with a diagnosis of early progressive idiopathic dementia (presumably of the Alzheimer's type) were treated with DDAVP (Weingartner et al. 1981b) in a crossover protocol. Significantly, the subjects were selected for high premorbid intellectual abilities and relatively minor deterioration. Peptide treatment improved performance on a task involving free verbal associations to letter or semantic category cues. These interesting results are encouraging, but the small number of subjects in each study and the inherent limitations in A-B-A and crossover designs make interpretations tentative.

Ferris et al. (in press) also used a crossover design to study the effects of LVP on 20 Alzheimer's disease subjects. Statistically significant improvement was found on memory tasks involving facial recognition, paired associate learning, and on a "carefree" factor of a self-rating mood scale. Positive trends were found on a reaction time task. Together, these results suggest nonspecific central nervous system stimulation. None of the changes, however, were clinically significant.

These relatively positive clinical studies should be examined in the context of other, less promising studies. Fourteen normal university students were treated for two weeks with either DDAVP or placebo in a parallel group study (Jenkins et al. 1982). There were no significant differences between the two groups. Several essentially negative trials of VP peptides have involved patients with cognitive deficits secondary to head trauma or alcoholism (Blake et al. 1978; Jenkins et al. 1979; Jenkins et al. 1981; Koch-Henriksen and Nielsen 1981; Reichert and Blass 1982; Tinklenberg et al. 1981; Tinklenberg et al. 1982a, 1982b; Tinklenberg et al., in press). Interpretations of these results should be limited because in each study subject samples were small. In addition, patients who were too impaired to respond to any intervention were probably included in some of these studies.

There have also been relatively unpromising reports of VP peptide treatment for primary degenerative dementia (presumably Alzheimer's disease). Three separate crossover studies using small numbers of quite impaired patients showed no significant peptide effects (Jenkins et al. 1982; Tinklenberg et al. 1981; Tinklenberg et al. 1982b). A larger scale parallel group study involved 14 subjects with Alzheimer's disease, seven of whom were treated with 16 IU of LVP intranasally for 10 days (Durso et al. 1982; Tamminga et al. 1982; Chase et al. 1982). The actively treated patients did not differ from the seven placebo subjects on learning and memory tasks, but they did show significantly faster fixed-interval reaction times during the course of the study. It is interesting that these faster responses persisted during post-treatment sessions. This persistent effect is compatible with prolonged VP activity in preclinical studies. In two pilot parallel group trials of DGAVP treatment, we have studied a total of 10 Alzheimer's patients (Tinklenberg et al. 1982a, in press). The five patients who received DGAVP treatment did not significantly differ from the placebo patients on learning and memory measures, although on several clinical scales the DGAVP-treated patients showed reductions in depression and increases in ratings of vigor.

Overall, these results suggest to us several themes regarding VP treatment in aging and dementia. (1) There are considerable discrepancies between the positive preclinical data and the inconsistent human findings. Possible reasons for these discrepancies are discussed below. (2) Most well-designed trials with severely impaired subjects have been negative. As noted in recent comprehensive reviews, there are anatomical and physiological reasons why VP peptides are not likely to be effective in people with extensive neuronal degeneration (Jolles, in press; Jolles et al., in press). (3) The most consistent clinical VP effects can be explained as nonspecific central nervous system stimulation and secondary changes in mood, attention, or other memory-modulating processes. This explanation is not as exciting as postulating that VP has direct effects on memory processes per se, but, if true, nevertheless does suggest that VP peptides may have a treatment role in certain geriatric disorders.

Other Neuropeptides

Other neuropeptides, such as the endorphins, enkephalins, melanocyte-inhibiting factor (MIF-1), and oxytocin, also influence animal behavior in certain conditions. Details and mechanisms of their effects appear to be complex (Belluzzi and Stein 1981; Izquierdo et al. 1981; Koob et al. 1981; Kovacs and De Wied 1981; Martinez et al. 1981; Messing et al. 1981; van Wimersma Greidanus et al. 1981). Initial human trials of these peptides have not focused on geriatric issues, but in the next few years a broader range of research questions are likely to be addressed. Naloxone, the inhibitor of endogenous opioid peptides, also affects behavior in animal studies (Messing et al. 1981).

A preliminary report of an open trial of naloxone in five patients with severe senile dementia of the Alzheimer's type is encouraging (Reisberg et al. 1983). None of the five patients tested demonstrated clinical or psychometric deterioration following naloxone injection. Two patients demonstrated clinically notable improvement, and one patient showed marked clinical improvement. Psychometric scores also indicated improvement in all patients who had demonstrated clinical response. Although the rationale for this potential effect is unclear, it may be that endogenous morphine-like substances, like exogenous morphine, impair attention and arousal; thus a narcotic antagonist such a naloxone might improve cognitive function if it could reduce the hypothesized attention impairment that endorphins might cause. Arnsten et al. (1973) recently reported that 2-mg naxolone injections enhanced selective attention in young men. Further work, including studies using active control drugs, is clearly indicated and will likely parallel the work already accomplished with VP and ACTH fragments.

Discrepancies Between Animal and Human Trials of Neuropeptides

The discrepancies between the results of nonhuman and human studies on the behavioral effects of neuropeptides highlight the difficulties in extrapolating from animal findings to clinical trials. One explanation for discrepant findings is that the designs of many human studies are not as rigorous or as appropriate as those in most animal studies (Gaillard 1981; Jolles, in press; Jolles et al., in press). In other words, if the correct clinical designs are used, the peptide effects found in animals will also be obtained in humans. An implication of this thesis is that clinical trials have not succeeded in combining the most advantageous mixture of such basic research variables as dosage, dose schedule, route of administration, and testing procedures. A second explanation for animal-human discrepancies in peptide studies is that the more complex psychological processes of humans are affected by different pharmacological variables than are the obviously simpler psychological processes of rodents and other laboratory animals (Rigter and Crabbe 1979). This thesis implies that if comparable paradigms are used, then the results of animal and human studies will be similar. Experiments designed to test this hypothesis have so far been negative (Miller et al. 1977). A third explanation for discrepant peptide findings in animal and human studies is that peptide-sensitive differences exist in critical anatomical and neurochemical substrates in different species and at different ages. Finally, there is probably more variability in response to a drug in humans of different genetic backgrounds and different life experiences over six or seven decades than there is between two-year-old rat littermates. Such increased variability makes it more difficult to document drug effects.

CONCLUDING COMMENTS

A considerable amount of evidence from nonhuman studies indicates that neuropeptides can exert significant behavioral effects. Some of the most consistent effects are observed in aged animals or animals that have impaired performance from hypophysectomy or other interventions. We feel that these positive behavioral effects probably result from nonspecific peptide activity, rather than from influences on specific memory functions.

Initial human trials of neuropeptide effects have produced less consistent results. Of the several possible explanations for the discrepancies between the positive animal findings and inconsistent human results, the most optimistic is that many human trials have used inappropriate designs. Inadequate dosage schedules, too-brief treatment periods, and excessively impaired subjects obviously hamper the proper evaluation of these peptides. Studies that employ larger peptide doses for longer periods of time with more appropriate patients are now being conducted. Such studies offer the possibility of overcoming most anatomical and neurochemical factors that limit availability of these peptides to the human central nervous system. Results from these trials should clarify the role of these peptides in geriatric psychopharmacology.

REFERENCES

Abuzzahab FS, Zimmermann RL, Will JC: ACTH 4–10 versus placebo in geriatric memory, in Proceedings of the Collegium Internationale Neuro-pharmacologicum Meeting. Vienna, Collegium Internationale Neuro-pharmacologicum, 1978

Arnstrn AFT, Segal DS, Neville HJ, et al: Naloxone augments electrophysiological signs of selective attention in man. Nature 304:725–727, 1983

Asin KE: Lysine vasopressin attenuation of diethyldithiocarbamate-induced amnesia. Pharmacol Biochem Behav 12:343–346, 1980

Barchas JD, Akil H, Elliott GR, et al: Behavioral neurochemistry: neuroregulators and behavioral states. Science 200:964–973, 1978

Belluzzi JD, Stein L: Facilitation of long-term memory by brain endorphins, in Endogenous Peptides and Learning and Memory Processes. Edited by Martinez J, Jensen RA, Messing RB, et al. New York, Academic Press, 1981

Berger PA, Tinklenberg JR: Neuropeptides and senile dementia, in Strategies for the Development of an Effective Treatment for Senile Dementia. Edited by Crook T, Gershon S. New Canaan, Conn, Mark Powley Associates Inc, 1981

Blake DR, Dodd MJ, Evans JG: Vasopressin in amnesia. Lancet 1:608, 1978

Bohus B: Effects of desglycinamine-lysine vasopressin (DG-LVP) on sexually motivated T-maze behavior of the male rat. Horm Behav 8:52–61, 1977

Bohus B, De Wied D: Actions of ACTH- and MSH-like peptides on learning, performance, and retention, in Endogenous Peptides and Learning and Memory Processes. Edited by Martinez J, Jensen RA, Messing RB, et al. New York, Academic Press, 1981

Bohus B, Gispen VH, De Wied D: Effects of lysine vasopressin and ACTH 4-10 on conditioned avoidance behavior of hypophysectomized rats. Neuroendocrinology 11:137–142, 1973

Bootin HB, Pffeiffer WD: Effect of lysine vasopressin on pentylenetetrazol-induced retrograde amnesia in rats. Pharmacol Biochem Behav 7:51–54, 1977

Branconnier RJ, Cole JO, Gardos G: ACTH 4–10 in the amelioration of neuropsychological symptomatology associated with senile organic brain syndrome. Psychopharmacology 61:161–165, 1979

Chase TN, Durso R, Fedio P, et al: Vasopressin treatment of cognitive deficits in Alzheimer's disease, in Alzheimer's Disease: A Report of Progress in Research. Edited by Corkin S, Davis KL, Growden JH, et al. New York, Raven Press, 1982

Cooper RL, McNamara MC, Thompson G: Vasopressin and conditioned flavor aversion in aged rats. Neurobiol Aging 1:53–57, 1980

De Wied D: Effects of peptide hormones on behavior, in Frontiers in Neuroendocrinology. Edited by Ganong WR, Martin K. New York, Oxford University Press, 1969

De Wied D: Long-term effect of vasopressin on the maintenance of a conditioned avoidance response in rats. Nature 232:58–60, 1971

De Wied D: Pituitary–adrenal system hormones and behavior, in The Neurosciences: Third Study Program. Edited by Schmitt FO, Worden FG. Cambridge, MIT Press, 1974

De Wied D: Behavioural actions of neurohypophysial peptides. Proc R Soc Lond [Biol] 210:183–195, 1980

De Wied D, Bohus B, van Wimersma Greidanus TJB: Memory deficit in rats with hereditary diabetes insipidus. Brain Res 85:152–156, 1975

Dornbush RL, Shapiro B, Freedman AM: Effects of an ACTH short chain neuropeptide in man. Am J Psychiatry 138:962–964, 1981

Dunn AJ, Gispen WH: How ACTH acts on the brain. Biobehavioral Reviews 1:15–23, 1977

Durso R, Fedio P, Brouwers P, et al: Lysine vasopressin in Alzheimer's disease. Neurology 32:674–677, 1982

Ferris SH, Gershon S: Our ACTH 4–9 study. Unpublished paper presented at the Meeting of the American College of Neuropsychopharmacology, San Juan, 1979

Ferris SH, Reisberg B, Schneck MK, et al: Effects of vasopressin on primary degenerative dementia, in Neuropeptide and Hormone Modulation of Brain Function and Homeostasis. Edited by Ordy JM, Sladek J, Reisberg B. New York, Raven Press (in press)

Ferris SH, Sathananathan G, Gershon S, et al: Cognitive effects of ACTH 4–10 in the elderly. Pharmacol Biochem Behav 5:73–78, 1976

Gaillard AWK: ACTH analogs and human performance, in Endogenous Peptides and Learning and Memory Processes. Edited by Martinez J, Jensen RA, Messing RB, et al. New York, Academic Press, 1981

Gold PW, Ballenger JC, Weingartner H, et al: Effects of 1-desamo-8-D-8-D-arginine vasopressin on behaviour and cognition in primary affective disorder. Lancet 2:992–994, 1979

Hostetter G, Jubb SL, Kolowski GP: Vasopressin affects the behavior of rats in a positively rewarded discrimination task. Life Sci 21:1323–1328, 1977

Izquierdo I, Perry ML, Dias RD, et al: Endogenous opioids, memory modulation, and state dependency, in Endogenous Peptides and Learning and Memory Processes. Edited by Martinez J, Jensen RA, Messing RB, et al. New York, Academic Press, 1981

Jenkins JS, Mather HM, Coughlan AD, et al: Desmopressin in posttraumatic amnesia. Lancet 2:1245–1246, 1979

Jenkins JS, Mather HM, Coughlan AD, et al: Desmopressin and desglycinamide vasopressin in posttraumatic amnesia. Lancet 1:39, 1981

Jenkins JS, Mather HM, Coughlan AD, et al: Effect of desmopressin on normal and impaired memory. J Neurol Neurosurg Psychiatry 45:830–831, 1982

Jolles J: Vasopressin-like peptides and the treatment of memory disorders in man, in Progress in Brain Research. Edited by Cross BA, Leng G. New York, Raven Press (in press)

Jolles J, Gaillard AWK, Hijman R: Memory disorders and vasopressin, in Proceedings of the Conference on Integrative Neurohumoral Mechanisms. Edited by Endroczi E. Amsterdam, Elsevier/North-Holland (in press)

Hunt EB, Tinklenberg JR: A methodology for studying the effects of drugs on human cognition: ACTH 4–9 analogue (Organon 2766) vs methylphenidate. Manuscript submitted for publication

Kastin AJ, Olson RD, Sandman CA, et al: Multiple independent actions of neuropeptides on behavior, in Endogenous Peptides and Learning and Memory Processes. Edited by Martinez J, Jensen RA, Messing RB, et al. New York, Academic Press, 1981

Koch-Henriksen N, Nielsen N: Vasopressin in post-traumatic amnesia. Lancet 1:38–39, 1981

Koob GF, Le Moal M, Bloom FE: Enkephalin and endorphin influences on appetitive and aversive conditioning, in Endogenous Peptides and Learning and Memory Processes. Edited by Martinez J, Jensen RA, Messing RB, et al. New York, Academic Press, 1981

Kovacs GL, De Wied D: Endorphin influences on learning and memory, in Endogenous Peptides and Learning and Memory Processes. Edited by Martinez J, Jensen RA, Messing RB, et al. New York, Academic Press, 1981

Krieger DT, Martin JB: Brain peptides (in two parts). N Engl J Med 304:876–885, 944–951, 1981

LeBoeuf A, Lodge J, Eames PG: Vasopressin and memory in Korsakoff's syndrome. Lancet 2:1370, 1978

Legros JJ, Gilot P, Seron X, et al: Influence of vasopressin on learning and memory. Lancet 1:41–42, 1978

Martinez J, Rigter H, Jensen RA, et al: Endorphin and enkephalin effects on avoidance conditioning: the other side of the pituitary-adrenal axis, in Endogenous Peptides and Learning and Memory Processes. Edited by Martinez J, Jensen RA, Messing RB, et al. New York, Academic Press, 1981

Messing RB, Jensen RA, Vasquez BJ, et al: Opiate modulation of memory, in Endogenous Peptides and Learning and Memory Processes. Edited by Martinez J, Jensen RA, Messing RB, et al. New York, Academic Press, 1981

Miller LH, Fischer SC, Groves GA, et al: MSH/ACTH 4-10 influences on the CAR in human subjects: a negative finding. Pharmacol Biochem Behav 7:417-419, 1977

Oliveros JC, Jandali MD, Timsit-Berthier M, et al: Vasopressin in amnesia. Lancet 1:42, 1978

Pigache RM: Effects of ACTH-like peptides on cognition and affect in the elderly, in Neuropeptide and Hormone Modulation of Brain Function and Homeostasis. Edited by Ordy JM, Sladek JR, Reisberg B. New York, Raven Press (in press[a])

Pigache RM: The human psychopharmacology of peptides related to ACTH and alpha-MSH, in Clinical Pharmacology and Psychiatry, vol 3. Edited by Gram L, Usdin E, Dahl S, et al. Basingstoke, England, Macmillan (in press[b])

Pigache RM: A peptide for the aged: basic and clinical studies, in Psychopharmacology of Old Age. Edited by Wheatley D. Oxford, Oxford University Press (in press[c])

Pigache RM, Rigter H: Effects of peptides related to ACTH on mood and vigilance in man. Frontiers of Hormone Research 8:193-207, 1981

Reichert WH, Blass JP: A placebo-controlled trial shows no effect of vasopressin on recovery from closed head injury. Ann Neurol 12:390-392, 1982

Reisberg B, Ferris SH, Anand R, et al: Naloxone effects on primary degenerative dementia (PDD). Psychopharmacol Bull 19:45–47, 1983

Rigter H: A peptide for the aged?—Animal Studies, in Psychopharmacology of Old Age. Edited by Wheatley D. Oxford, Oxford University Press (in press)

Rigter H, Crabbe JC: Modulation of memory by pituitary hormones and related peptides. Vitam Horm 37:153–241, 1979

Rigter H, van Riezen H: Pituitary hormones and amnesia, in Current Developments in Psychopharmacology, vol 5. Edited by Essman WB, Valzelli L. New York, Spectrum Publications, 1979

Rigter H, Elbutse R, van Riezen H: Time dependent antiamnesia effects of ACTH 4–10 and desglycinamide-lysine vasopressin. Prog Brain Res 42:163–171, 1975

Rigter H, van Riezen H, De Wied D: The effects of ACTH and vasopressin analogues on CO_2-induced retrograde amnesia in rats. Physiol Behav 13:381–388, 1974

Sandman CA, Kastin AJ: Pituitary peptide influences on attention and memory, in Neurobiology of Sleep and Memory. Edited by Drucker-Colin RR, McGaugh JL. New York, Academic Press, 1977

Sandman CA, Alexander WD, Kastin AJ: Neuroendocrine influences on visual discrimination and reversal learning in the albino and hooded rats. Physiol Behav 11:613–617, 1973

Tamminga CA, Durso R, Fedio P, et al: Vasopressin studies in Alzheimer's disease. Psychopharmacol Bull 18:48–49, 1982

Tinklenberg JR, Peabody CA, Berger PA: Vasopressin effects on cognition and affect in the elderly, in Neuropeptide and Hormone Modulation of Brain Function and Homeostasis. Edited by Ordy JM, Sladek JR, Reisberg B. New York, Raven Press (in press.)

Tinklenberg JR, Pfefferbaum A, Berger PA: 1-Desamino-D-arginine vasopressin (DDAVP) in cognitively impaired patients. Psychopharmacol Bull 17:206–207, 1981

Tinklenberg JR, Pigache RM, Berger PA, et al: Desglycinamide-9-arginine-8-vasopressin (DGAVP, Organon 5667) in cognitively impaired patients. Psychopharmacol Bull 18:202–204, 1982a

Tinklenberg JR, Pigache RM, Pfefferbaum A, et al: Vasopressin peptides and dementia, in Alzheimer's Disease: A Report of Progress in Research. Vol 19. Edited by Corkin S, Davis KL, Growdon JH, et al. New York, Raven Press, 1982b

van Wimersma Greidanus TB: Effects of MSH and related peptides on avoidance behavior in rats. Frontiers of Hormonal Research 4:129–133, 1977

van Wimersma Greidanus TB, Bohus B, De Wied D: Vasopressin and oxytocin in learning and memory, in Endogenous Peptides and Learning and Memory Processes. Edited by Martinez J, Jensen RA, Messing RB, et al. New York, Academic Press, 1981

van Wimersma Greidanus TB, Dogterom J, De Wied D: Intraventricular administration of anti-vasopressin serum inhibits memory consolidation in rats. Life Sci 16:637–644, 1975

Versteeg DHG: Interaction of peptides related to ACTH, MSH, and beta-LPH with neurotransmitters in the brain. Pharmacol Ther 11:535–557, 1980

Weingartner H, Gold P, Ballenger JC, et al: Effects of vasopressin on human memory functions. Science 211:601–603, 1981a

Weingartner H, Kaye W, Gold P, et al: Vasopressin treatment of cognitive dysfunction in progressive dementia. Life Sci 29:2721–2726, 1981b

Witter A, Gispen WH, De Wied D: Mechanisms of action of behaviorally active ACTH-like peptides, in Endogenous Peptides and Learning and Memory Processes. Edited by Martinez J, Jensen RA, Messing RB, et al. New York, Academic Press, 1981

7

Biologic Parameters in the Differential Diagnosis of Dementia and Depression

Murray Raskind, M.D.

7

Biologic Parameters in the Differential Diagnosis of Dementia and Depression

The two most frequent psychiatric disorders of later life, depression and dementia, have several signs and symptoms in common. Impaired cognitive function, the essential feature of dementia, frequently occurs in late-life depression. On the other hand, several major signs and symptoms of depression, including loss of interest in the environment, agitation or retardation, sleep disturbance, and appetite disturbance, frequently occur in dementing illnesses. This overlap of signs and symptoms between depression and dementia presents the clinician with problems in differential diagnosis. In the extreme case, a depressed patient can be so cognitively impaired that his or her clinical presentation mimics dementia. Such "depressive pseudodementia" can usually be recognized as depression with prominent cognitive impairment on the basis of a careful history, mental status examination, and clinical observation (Wells 1979). In exceptional cases, however, the true nature of the illness will remain elusive. An even more difficult diagnostic problem, and one that is more common than "depressive pseudodementia," is the recognition of a depressive disorder complicating a clearly present dementing illness (Reifler et al. 1982). Such "secondary" depressions can compromise the demented patient's already impaired cognitive and behavioral function. Because data obtained from the clinical interview of the forgetful and sometimes aphasic dementia patient can be difficult to interpret, the recognition of a coexistent depression can be obscured.

Given these diagnostic problems, objective biological parameters that could help separate depression and dementia would be useful. Neuroendocrine measures, particularly the dexamethasone suppression test (DST) (Carroll et al. 1981), and sleep parameters, particularly REM latency (Kupfer et al. 1981), are frequently abnormal in depression. Neuroradiographic measures, particularly computed tomographic (CT) scanning (Jacoby and Levy 1980a), appear to be abnormal in dementing illnesses. Therefore, these biological parameters may have clinical utility in the differential diagnosis of depression and dementia.

This chapter will review evidence supporting the presence of cognitive impairment in dementia and the prevalence of depression in dementing illnesses. It will then review the applicability of the DST, sleep parameters, and the CT scan to the clinical task of teasing apart depression and dementia in the elderly patient.

PRESENCE OF DEPRESSION IN DEMENTIA PATIENTS

Several early clinical studies of dementia and depression in the elderly drew attention to the frequency with which dementia patients exhibited signs and symptoms of depression. Serious suicidal tendencies and profound as well as convincingly communicated depressions occur in demented patients, and depressed dementia patients have a suicide risk as high as elderly depressed patients without evidence of dementia (Post 1972). In one study, 50 percent of elderly patients who attempted suicide were suffering from dementia or delirium (O'Neal et al. 1956). Another study found evidence of depression in 56 percent of mildly demented patients and in 25 percent of severely demented patients (Ernst et al. 1977). A recent, well-designed study (Miller 1980) documented a high frequency of depressive symptomatology in patients with dementia of the Alzheimer's type. Dementia patients without previously identified depression had a mean score of 16 on the Hamilton Psychiatric Rating Scale for Depression (Hamilton

1960), which falls into the mild-to-moderately depressed range. Although the mean Hamilton score was lower in demented patients than in nondemented elderly depressed patients (25.98), it was significantly higher than the mean Hamilton score in normal elderly persons (4.97). Even more striking evidence for depression in the dementia patients was demonstrated by the scores on the Beck Depression Inventory (Beck et al. 1961). On this self-rated scale, the depressed nondemented patients' mean score of 11.43 was not significantly different from the demented patients' mean score of 9.74. In contrast, the mean Beck Depression Inventory score for the normal elderly group was 2.90. Thus, patients with mild-to-moderate dementia had an unexpectedly high level of depressive symptomatology. It was of further interest that the families of many of the dementia patients reported that these dysphoric mood states had often persisted for many months.

IMPAIRMENT OF COGNITION IN DEPRESSION

The predominance of evidence concerning the effect of depression on cognition indicates that depression per se impairs cognitive function. An early study (Rapaport 1945) indicated that depressed patients performed poorly on the Wechsler Adult Intelligence Scale and on a digit span and story recall test. Depressed patients also performed more poorly than controls at reproducing learned material (Cronholm and Ottoson 1961). In a recent, carefully designed study (Weingartner et al. 1981), depressed patients demonstrated both qualitative and quantitative changes in information processing, leading to impaired memory. The most convincing evidence that depression reversibly impairs cognitive function comes from studies of improvement in cognitive function following successful treatment of depressed patients. Improvement in the learning of new material and in psychomotor speed has been documented in elderly depressed patients following treatment with either the tricyclic antidepressant, amitriptyline, or electroconvulsive therapy (Cawley et al. 1973). The small subgroups of patients with depression superimposed upon dementia showed similar improvement to that of the larger group of nondemented depressed patients. Impaired performance on serial and free recall verbal learning tasks during depression improved after treatment with the psychoactive drugs L-dopa and L-tryptophan (Henry et al. 1973). Impaired memory function as measured by the Wechsler Memory Scale was documented in depressed patients, and recovery from depression following unilateral electroconvulsive therapy eliminated the memory impairment (Stromgren 1977). Marked deficits in short-term memory in depressed patients have also improved following successful treatment with imipramine (Sternberg and Jarvik 1976). In summary, most clinical studies suggest that depression impairs cognitive function, particularly short-term memory and strategies of information processing, and that these cognitive deficits improve following effective treatment of the patient's depression.

THE DEXAMETHASONE SUPPRESSION TEST

A large body of experimental data supports the hypothesis that early escape of plasma cortisol from suppression by dexamethasone differentiates endogenous depression or melancholia from other psychiatric illnesses, at least in the inpatient population. Approximately 50 percent of endogenously depressed inpatients will have a plasma cortisol greater than 5 μg/dl during the 24-hour period following a 1-mg dose of dexamethasone ingested late the previous evening (Carroll et al. 1981). It has therefore been suggested that a positive DST (early escape of plasma cortisol from dexamethasone suppression) would favor the diagnosis of depression over dementia in the cognitively impaired patient. Evidence supporting this suggestion has been derived primarily from case reports. A 64-year-old woman with mild cognitive impairment and a clinical picture compatible with endogenous depression had a positive DST which reverted to normal (along with her cognitive impairment) after a course of tricyclic antidepressant therapy (Rudorfer and Clayton 1981). Although this case is interesting as an illustration of reversible cognitive impairment in the severely depressed patient, it is unlikely that many clinicians would have had difficulty diagnosing this patient's depression even in the absence of a positive DST. Another report described two patients with severe cognitive impairment and positive DSTs, both of whom responded to either electroconvulsive therapy or tricyclic antidepressant therapy (McAllister et al. 1982). In the first patient, a 75-year-old woman with significant underlying medical illness and weight loss, the DST reverted to normal following treatment. Although cognitive function improved, she continued to have some cognitive dysfunction. In the second patient, a 72-year-old man with positive neurologic signs and probably cerebral infarctions on CT scan, the DST remained abnormal despite marked improvement in both mood and cognitive function. These cases appear to represent patients with underlying dementing illnesses and secondary depression rather than true depressive pseudodementia, and illustrate how a superimposed depression can reversibly impair cognitive function in the patient with underlying structural brain disease.

An important report carefully described five patients in whom communication deficits secondary to extensive structural brain damage masked the presence of treatable depression (Ross and Rush 1981). In three of these instructive patients the DST was positive, and in two patients in whom antidepressant therapy was successful, the DST normalized following improvement in affective status. These investigators interpreted their findings as illustrative of the value of the DST as a biological marker in establishing the existence of depression in brain-damaged patients. It should be noted that in both patients in whom the DST normalized, it was positive in the context of severe weight loss and returned to normal in association with significant weight gain. In the third DST-positive patient, marked anorexia was mentioned, but weight was not described and the patient's deteriorating cardiac and cerebral vascular status precluded antidepressant therapy. Although DST abnormalities in these patients may have been unrelated to weight loss, it should be mentioned that weight loss alone has been associated with a positive DST in the absence of depression or other psychiatric or medical illness (Edelstein et al. 1983).

DST results in a more extensive series of patients with signs and symptoms of both depression and dementia have been reported (Grunhaus et al. 1983). These 11 patients received both a DST and a CT scan as part of their diagnostic evaluations. Eight of the 11 patients had positive DSTs. Although the retrospective nature of this study and the small number of patients evaluated (particularly in the DST-negative group) limited definitive interpretation, these investigators found that patients with a positive DST, particularly in the presence of a normal CT scan, appeared more likely to improve in both depressive symptomatology and cognitive dysfunction than patients with a negative DST. They proposed a model in which a profile of three elements (the diagnosis of a major depressive disorder, a positive DST, and a normal CT scan) suggests the diagnosis of depressive pseudodementia. They further proposed that this model be tested in prospective studies.

Before the DST can be accepted as a valid diagnostic tool for the differentiation of depression from dementia, it must first be demonstrated that dementing illnesses per se, particularly Alzheimer's disease and multi-infarct dementia, are not associated with a positive DST. It is also necessary to rule out that advanced age is associated with a positive DST. If either dementia or advanced age is associated with a positive DST, then the specificity of the DST as a marker for depression in this population will be lost. At this time, advanced age does not appear to be associated with an increased rate of positive DSTs, at least as standardized for use in psychiatric patients (1 mg of dexamethasone given at 11:00 P.M., followed by blood cortisol determinations at 4:00 P.M. and 11:00 P.M. the next day). There is no significant difference in either cortisol circadian rhythm or cortisol response to the standard DST in young versus elderly medically and psychiatrically healthy populations (Turigny-Rivard et al. 1981).

Unfortunantely, recent reports suggest that dementing illnesses themselves are associated with an increased incidence of positive DST results. The DST was administered to elderly demented patients who were hospitalized for evaluation and treatment (Spar and Gerner 1982). Nine of 17 demented patients, all of whom were free of major depressive disorder, had a positive DST. Patients with Alzheimer's disease, multi-infarct dementia, and dementia secondary to Parkinson's disease were included in the DST-positive group. Although the DST-positive group was somewhat older than the DST-negative group, the severity of dementia—predominatly mild or moderate as measured by the Mini-Mental State (Folstein et al. 1975)—did not differ between the two groups. A control population was not included in this study. These findings were extended by another study (Raskind et al. 1982). These investigators administered the standardized DST to 15 inpatients with advanced Alzheimer's disease and to 15 age-matched normal controls. Both groups were free of a depressive disorder. Seven of the 15 patients with advanced Alzheimer's disease were DST-positive as compared to none of the normal controls. The 47 percent rate of DST nonsuppression in the Alzheimer's patients was similar to that described in non-demented patients with endogenous depression. These results confirmed that a positive DST is common in nondepressed dementia patients and cast further doubt on the utility of the DST in the diagnosis of depression complicating advanced dementia.

Similar findings were reported in a group of mildly to moderately demented outpatients suffering from either Alzheimer's disease or multi-infarct dementia (Balldin et al. 1983). Twelve of 21 Alzheimer's disease patients and eight of 11 multi-infarct dementia patients were DST positive compared with just one of 14 healthy age-matched controls. Yet another study has reported similar findings (Davis et al. 1983). These investigators administered standard DST to 18 Alzheimer's disease patients, all of whom were ambulatory and physically healthy, and most of whom were still living at home. None of these patients met DSM-III criteria for depression. Nine of the 18 patients had a positive DST, and all Alzheimer's patients with an onset of illness over age 65 had a positive DST. Neither severity of dementia nor incidence of depressive symptoms differentiated positive DST patients from negative DST patients. Only one published study has found normal DST results in dementia patients (Carnes et al. 1983). The investigators administered the standard DST to seven Alzheimer's disease patients and five multi-infarct dementia patients. None of these 12 patients were DST positive. The mean age of these patients (80.2 years) was significantly higher than the mean ages in the other studies of the DST in dementia, and these patients were generally mildly demented.

Taken together, these studies of the DST in dementia patients raise serious questions concerning the value of this test in the differential diagnosis of depression and dementia. If a positive DST can be associated with either depression or dementia, the clinician derives little benefit from the DST as a biological marker in differentiating these two illnesses. On the other hand, the DST may be useful in longitudinal management of the individual patient with either depressive pseudodementia or depression complicating a dementing disorder. If the DST changes from positive to negative after antidepressant treatment (provided that significant weight loss was not present at the time the DST was positive), this finding would retroactively support the diagnosis of a reversible depression. How much more this information would add to data derived from standard clinical evaluation, however, remains to be determined by prospective studies.

SLEEP PARAMETERS

All-night electroencephalographic recordings have revealed consistent abnormalities in patients with major depressive disorders. Particularly striking have been changes involving REM sleep. Of these changes, shortened REM latency (the time between sleep onset and the beginning of the first REM period minus time awake) has been particularly consistent across studies (Kupfer 1976). The phenomenon of decreased REM latency in major depressive disorder does not appear to be altered by advanced age (Kupfer et al. 1978; Reynolds et al., 1980). If REM latency is not shortened by dementing disorders, this potential biologic marker could prove useful in the separation of depression and dementia. REM sleep parameters were studied in nine mild, nine moderate, and nine severe Alzheimer's disease subjects and in nine age-matched normal controls (Vitiello et al. in press). All subjects were free of major depressive disorder. Results indicated that REM sleep measures were minimally affected by mild dementia. Of particular importance was the finding that REM latency as measured by time from sleep onset to first REM period minus intervening wake time did not significantly differ between normal controls and any stage of dementing illness. If anything, the demented patients showed a tendency toward prolongation of REM latency. Another group retrospectively compared the sleep recordings of nine patients with primary degenerative dementia by DSM-III criteria (a diagnosis compatible with Alzheimer's disease) to those of nine age-matched patients with major depressive disorder (Reynolds et al. 1983). Subjects were also matched as to age and inpatient or outpatient status. Depressed patients had a higher density of rapid eye movements during REM sleep and less sleep-continuity disturbance than did dementia patients. Although REM sleep was shorter in the depressed patients, the difference was not statistically significant. Using a cutoff score of 30 minutes for REM latency, 14 of 18 patients were correctly classified. Six of nine depressed patients (67 percent) had a REM latency less than 30 minutes, and eight of nine dementia patients (89 percent) had a REM latency of 30 minutes or more.

Taken together, these studies of sleep parameters in dementia and depression suggest that REM latency and other sleep parameters may prove to be useful biologic markers in the differential diagnosis of depression and dementia. Although sleep studies are more difficult to perform than neuroendocrine studies such as the DST, sleep laboratories are becoming increasingly commonplace. More and larger prospective studies of sleep parameters in elderly depressed and demented patients clearly need to be performed.

COMPUTED TOMOGRAPHY

The advent of the computed tomographic (CT) scan has provided a safe and noninvasive means of examining intracranial content. Such technology has raised the possibility that CT scan findings of ventricular dilatation, sulcal widening, and decreased brain density might help establish the diagnosis of dementia. If dementia patients can be truly separated from normal elderly persons and from elderly persons suffering from "functional" psychiatric disorders using these parameters, then the CT scan would be a helpful biologic marker in the differential diagnosis of dementia and depression (Grunhaus et al. 1983). Studies addressing this problem have yielded mixed results. CT parameters of ventricular size and cortical atrophy were studied in 50 normal elderly subjects and 40 patients with senile dementia (Alzheimer's disease) (Jacoby and Levy 1980b). The senile dementia subjects showed significantly more CT evidence of cerebral atrophy than did the normal subjects, but unfortunately there was considerable overlap. Another study compared CT findings in 57 patients with senile dementia of the Alzheimer's type, 19 patients with multi-infarct dementia, and 85 normal controls of similar age and sex (Soininen et al. 1982). The Alzheimer's patients differed from the controls in ventricular dilatation, frontal horn index, width of the third ventricle, and a sulcal index of cortical atrophy. Even the least severely demented Alzheimer's patient group differed from the normal controls. The multi-infarct dementia patients also differed from controls in all CT variables, including focal changes. Again, however, there was some overlap in CT parameter values of dementia patients and normal elderly controls in individual cases, particularly in early stages of dementia. Another study examined CT scans of patients with senile dementia of the Alzheimer's type and age-matched normal controls (Wilson et al. 1982). Although dementia patients showed significantly more atrophy than controls, there was a great degree of overlap between the two groups. CT scan parameters have been examined in patients with presenile-onset Alzheimer's disease and were found to be helpful in discriminating patients from age-matched normal controls (Naeser et al. 1982). The most powerful measures in this regard were the volume of the bodies of the lateral ventricles. Linear measurements were useful, but not as discriminating.

Several investigators have also used CT scan technology to evaluate brain density in Alzheimer's disease. Mean CT numbers of Hounsfield units in 15 brain regions in routine CT scans were compared in 25 patients with senile dementia of the Alzheimer's type and 29 normal, community volunteer controls (Bondareff et al. 1981). These density measurements were significantly lower bilaterally in the medial temporal lobe, anterior frontal lobe, and head of the caudate nucleus in the demented patients than in controls. Another study reported that CT density measured in the centrum semiovale could separate demented patients from controls without overlap (Naeser et al. 1980). On the other hand, some investigators found CT density measures were no different between dementia patients and controls (Wilson et al. 1982). To complicate matters further, even though depression is a "functional" psychiatric illness, there have been reports of CT scan abnormalities in this disorder (Jacoby and Levy 1980a, 1980b; Pearlson and Veroff 1981). It therefore appears that before CT scan parameters can be accepted as specific for dementia in comparison with depression, larger studies evaluating standardized CT scan parameters will have to be performed. At present it appears that overlap of CT scan parameters between demented subjects and normal elderly patients limits the clinical utility of CT scan parameters in the differential diagnosis of dementia and depression.

SUMMARY

The diagnostic dilemma of the separation of depression and dementia is probably still best resolved by a careful history and clinical examination. The DST appears too nonspecific to be very useful in these populations. Sleep parameters, particularly REM latency, hold promise but have not yet been prospectively studied in large numbers of patients. CT scan parameters may prove useful, but present findings are too conflicting to recommend the CT scan as a reliable differential diagnostic technique. Larger studies including both demented and depressed patients, however, may define a differential diagnostic role for the CT scan. For the clinician, if doubt remains as to the true nature of the diagnosis, and signs and symptoms of depression are present, a cautious but determined trial of antidepressant therapy is warranted and may greatly benefit the patient. It must be borne in mind, however, that the adverse effects of many antidepressant drugs can sometimes outweigh any improvement in affective status and can actually be detrimental to the demented patient in whom a depressive disorder is not present.

References

Balldin J, Gottfries CG, Karlsson I, et al: Dexamethasone suppression test and serum prolactin in dementia disorders. Br J Psychiatry 143:277–281, 1983

Beck AT, Ward CH, Mendelson M, et al: An inventory for measuring depression. Arch Gen Psychiatry 4:561–571, 1961

Bondareff W, Baldy R, Levy R: Quantitative computed tomography in senile dementia. Arch Gen Psychiatry 38:1365–1368, 1981

Carnes M, Smith JC, Kalin NH, et al: Effects of chronic medical illness and dementia on the dexamethasone suppression test. J Am Geriatr Soc 31:269–271, 1983

Carroll BJ, Feinberg M, Greden JF, et al: A specific laboratory test for the diagnosis of melancholia. Arch Gen Psychiatry 38:15–22, 1981

Cawley RH, Post F, Whitehead A: Barbiturate tolerance and psychological functioning in elderly depressed patients. Psychol Med 3:39–52, 1973

Cronholm B, Ottoson JO: Memory functions in endogenous depression before and after electroconvulsive therapy. Arch Gen Psychiatry 5:193–199, 1961

Davis KL, Davis BM, Greenwald BS, et al: Hypercortisolemia in Alzheimer's disease. Presented at the 136th Annual Meeting of the American Psychiatric Association, New York, May 1983

Edelstein CK, Roy-Byrne P, Fawzy FI, et al: Effects of weight loss on the dexamethasone suppression test. Am J Psychiatry 140:338–341, 1983

Ernst P, Badash D, Berzan B, et al: Incidence of mental illness in the aged. J Am Geriatr Soc 25:371–375, 1977

Folstein MF, Folstein SE, McHugh PR: "Mini-mental state," a practical method for grading the cognitive state of patients for the clinician. J Psychiatr Res 12:189–197, 1975

Grunhaus L, Dilsaver S, Greden JF, et al: Depressive pseudodementia: a suggested diagnostic profile. Biol Psychiatry 18:215–225, 1983

Hamilton M: A rating scale for depression. J Neurol Neurosurg Psychiatry 23:56–62, 1960

Henry GM, Weingartner H, Murphy DL: Influence of affective states and psychoactive drugs on verbal learning and memory. Am J Psychiatry 130:966–971, 1973

Jacoby RJ, Levy R: Computed tomography in the elderly, II: senile dementia: diagnosis and functional impairment. Br J Psychiatry 136:256–269, 1980b

Jacoby RJ, Levy R, Dawson JN: Computed tomography in the elderly, I: normal population. Br J Psychiatry 136:249–255, 1980a

Kupfer DJ: REM latency: a psychobiologic marker for primary depressive disease. Biol Psychiatry 11:159–164, 1976

Kupfer DJ, Spiker DG, Coble PA, et al: Electroencephalographic sleep recordings and depression in the elderly. J Am Geriatr Soc 26:53–57, 1978

Kupfer DJ, Spiker DG, Coble PA, et al: Sleep and treatment prediction in endogenous depression. Am J Psychiatry 138:429–434, 1981

McAllister TW, Ferrell RB, Price TRP, et al: The dexamethasone suppression test in two patients with severe depressive pseudodementia. Am J Psychiatry 139:479–481, 1982

Miller NE: The measurement of mood in senile brain disease: exam ratings and self reports, in Psychopathology of the Aged. Edited by Cole JO, Barrett JE. New York, Raven Press, 1980, pp 97–118

Nazer MA, Albert MS, Levine H, Garvey J: CT scans: evaluation of patients with presenile dementia. Presented at the 35th Annual Meeting of the Gerontological Society, G Boston, November 1982

O'Neal P, Robins E, Schmidt EH: A psychiatric study of attempted suicide in persons over 60 years of age. Archives of Neurology and Psychiatry 75:275–279, 1956

Pearlson GD, Veroff AE: Computed tomographic scan changes in manic depressive illness. Lancet 2:470, 1981

Post F: The management and nature of depressive illness in late life. Br J Psychiatry 121:393–404, 1972

Rapaport P: Diagnostic Psychological Testing. Chicago, Year Book Medical Publishers, 1945

Raskind M, Peskind E, Rivard ME, et al: Dexamethasone suppression test and cortisol circadian rhythm in primary degenerative dementia. Am J Psychiatry 139:1468–1471, 1982

Reifler BV, Larson E, Hanley R: Coexistence of cognitive impairment and depression in geriatric outpatients. Am J Psychiatry 139:623–629, 1982

Reynolds CF, Coble PA, Black RS, et al: Sleep disturbances in a series of elderly patients: polysomnographic findings. J Am Geriatr Soc 28:164–170, 1980

Reynolds CF, Spiker DG, Hanin I: Electroencephalographic sleep, aging, and psychopathology: new data and state of the art. Biol Psychiatry 18:139–155, 1983

Ross ED, Rush AJ: Diagnosis and neuroanatomical correlates of depression in brain-damaged patients. Arch Gen Psychiatry 38:1344–1354, 1981

Rudorfer MV, Clayton PV: Depression, dementia, and dexamethasone suppression (ltr to ed). Am J Psychiatry 138:701, 1981

Soininen H, Puranen M, Riekinnen PJ: Computed tomography findings in senile dementia and normal aging. J Neurol Neurosurg Psychiatry 45:50–54, 1982

Spar JE, Gerner R: Does the dexamethasone suppression test distinguish dementia from depression? Am J Psychiatry 139:238–240, 1982

Sternberg DE, Jarvik ME: Memory functions in depression: improvement with antidepressant medication. Arch Gen Psychiatry 33:219–224, 1976

Stromgren LS: The influence of depression on memory. Acta Psychiatr Scand 56:109–128, 1977

Turigny-Rivard MF, Raskind MA, Rivard D: The dexamethasone suppression test in an elderly population. Biol Psychiatry 16:1177–1184, 1981

Vitiello MV, Bokan JA, Kukull WA, et al: Rapid eye movement sleep measures of Alzheimer's type dementia patients and optimally healthy aged individuals. Biol Psychiatry (in press)

Weingartner H, Cohen RM, Murphy DL, et al: Cognitive processes in depression. Arch Gen Psychiatry 38:42–47, 1981

Wells CE: Pseudodementia. Am J Psychiatry 136:895–900, 1979

Wilson RS, Fox JH, Huckman MS, et al: Computed tomography in dementia. Neurology 32:1054–1057, 1982